Nikolaos Pagonas

External counterpulsation: a novel therapy to stimulate arteriogenesis

Nikolaos Pagonas

External counterpulsation: a novel therapy to stimulate arteriogenesis

Südwestdeutscher Verlag für Hochschulschriften

Impressum/Imprint (nur für Deutschland/only for Germany)
Bibliografische Information der Deutschen Nationalbibliothek: Die Deutsche Nationalbibliothek verzeichnet diese Publikation in der Deutschen Nationalbibliografie; detaillierte bibliografische Daten sind im Internet über http://dnb.d-nb.de abrufbar.
Alle in diesem Buch genannten Marken und Produktnamen unterliegen warenzeichen-, marken- oder patentrechtlichem Schutz bzw. sind Warenzeichen oder eingetragene Warenzeichen der jeweiligen Inhaber. Die Wiedergabe von Marken, Produktnamen, Gebrauchsnamen, Handelsnamen, Warenbezeichnungen u.s.w. in diesem Werk berechtigt auch ohne besondere Kennzeichnung nicht zu der Annahme, dass solche Namen im Sinne der Warenzeichen- und Markenschutzgesetzgebung als frei zu betrachten wären und daher von jedermann benutzt werden dürften.

Verlag: Südwestdeutscher Verlag für Hochschulschriften GmbH & Co. KG
Dudweiler Landstr. 99, 66123 Saarbrücken, Deutschland
Telefon +49 681 37 20 271-1, Telefax +49 681 37 20 271-0
Email: info@svh-verlag.de

Approved by: Berlin, Charité-Universitätsmedizin, Diss., 2011

Herstellung in Deutschland:
Schaltungsdienst Lange o.H.G., Berlin
Books on Demand GmbH, Norderstedt
Reha GmbH, Saarbrücken
Amazon Distribution GmbH, Leipzig
ISBN: 978-3-8381-2741-5

Imprint (only for USA, GB)
Bibliographic information published by the Deutsche Nationalbibliothek: The Deutsche Nationalbibliothek lists this publication in the Deutsche Nationalbibliografie; detailed bibliographic data are available in the Internet at http://dnb.d-nb.de.
Any brand names and product names mentioned in this book are subject to trademark, brand or patent protection and are trademarks or registered trademarks of their respective holders. The use of brand names, product names, common names, trade names, product descriptions etc. even without a particular marking in this works is in no way to be construed to mean that such names may be regarded as unrestricted in respect of trademark and brand protection legislation and could thus be used by anyone.

Publisher: Südwestdeutscher Verlag für Hochschulschriften GmbH & Co. KG
Dudweiler Landstr. 99, 66123 Saarbrücken, Germany
Phone +49 681 37 20 271-1, Fax +49 681 37 20 271-0
Email: info@svh-verlag.de

Printed in the U.S.A.
Printed in the U.K. by (see last page)
ISBN: 978-3-8381-2741-5

Copyright © 2011 by the author and Südwestdeutscher Verlag für Hochschulschriften GmbH & Co. KG and licensors
All rights reserved. Saarbrücken 2011

Dedicated to my parents

Table of Contents

1 **INTRODUCTION** 5
   1.1   CORONARY ARTERY DISEASE 5
      1.1.1   *Epidemiology* 5
      1.1.2   *Pathophysiology* 5
      1.1.3   *Clinical features of stable coronary disease* 6
      1.1.4   *Diagnostic tests* 7
      1.1.5   *Therapy for stable CAD* 9
   1.2   ARTERIOGENESIS 11
      1.2.1   *Terminology of vascular growth* 11
      1.2.2   *Collateral artery growth and the role of shear stress* 12
      1.2.3   *The protective role of coronary collateral circulation* 15
      1.2.4   *Assessment of cardiac collateral arteries* 16
      1.2.5   *Clinical trials for the stimulation of arteriogenesis* 18
   1.3   EXTERNAL COUNTERPULSATION 19
      1.3.1   *Introduction* 19
      1.3.2   *Technique of ECP* 20
      1.3.3   *Mechanism of the action and review of the literature* 22

2 **THE STUDY'S HYPOTHESIS** 29

3 **PATIENTS AND METHODS** 30
   3.1   STUDY POPULATION 30
      3.1.1   *Inclusion and exclusion criteria* 30
   3.2   THE STUDY DESIGN 31
   3.3   CLINICAL ENDPOINTS AND NON-INVASIVE MEASUREMENTS 34
      3.3.1   *History and clinical examination* 34
      3.3.2   *Clinical laboratory evaluation* 35
      3.3.3   *Exercise test* 35
      3.3.4   *Cardiac magnetic resonance imaging* 35
   3.4   INVASIVE MEASUREMENTS AND ENDPOINTS 36
      3.4.1   *Fractional Flow Reserve (FFR)* 36
      3.4.2   *Collateral flow index (CFIp)* 38
      3.4.3   *Index of microcirculatory resistance (IMR)* 40
      3.4.4   *Quantitative coronary angiography* 42
      3.4.5   *Protocol of cardiac catheterization and invasive measurements* 42
      3.4.6   *Performance of the invasive measurements* 43
      3.4.7   *Calculation of the invasive endpoints* 44
   3.5   EXTERNAL COUNTERPULSATION THERAPY (ECP) 45
   3.6   SAMPLE SIZE AND STATISTICAL ANALYSIS 45

4 RESULTS 47
4.1 PATIENTS 47
4.1.1 Characteristics of the study population 47
4.1.2 Adverse events and compliance 49
4.2 ENDPOINTS AT BASELINE 49
4.2.1 Clinical characteristics of the patients 49
4.2.2 Hemodynamic effect of ECP 51
4.2.3 Non-invasive diagnostic tests at baseline 51
4.2.4 Invasive endpoints at baseline 53
4.3 ENDPOINTS AT WEEK 8 56
4.3.1 Clinical endpoints 56
4.3.2 Specific hemodynamic parameters 58
4.3.3 Exercise test 60
4.3.4 CMR 61
4.3.5 Invasive measurements 61
4.3.6 Univariate analysis 64

5 DISCUSSION 65
5.1 ESTABLISHMENT AND FEASIBILITY OF THE THERAPY 65
5.2 CLINICAL BENEFIT OF ECP 66
5.3 EXERCISE TEST AND ECP 68
5.4 ECP, ARTERIOGENESIS AND MYOCARDIAL BLOOD FLOW 69
5.4.1 Stimulation of arteriogenesis by ECP 69
5.4.2 ECP compared to pharmacologic stimulation of arteriogenesis 70
5.4.3 Collateral and myocardial blood flow 71
5.4.4 Clinical impact of ECP treatment 72
5.4.5 New data on the mechanism of action of ECP 72
5.4.6 Effectiveness ratio and response to the therapy 74
5.5 EFFECT ON CORONARY MICROCIRCULATION 75
5.5.1 Hemodynamic aspects of IMR 75
5.6 EFFECT OF ECP ON THE LEFT VENTRICULAR FUNCTION 76
5.7 LIMITATIONS OF THE STUDY 77

6 REFERENCES 78

7 APPENDIX 91
7.1 LIST OF ABBREVIATIONS 91
7.2 ACKNOWLEDGMENTS 93

1 Introduction

1.1 Coronary artery disease

1.1.1 Epidemiology

Cardiovascular disease is one of the industrial world's leading causes of death and morbidity. In Germany it accounted for about 364.000 deaths in 2008. Among cardiovascular diseases, ischemic heart disease is the leading cause of death and accounts for about 64% of the deaths. Most people (91%) who die from a cardiovascular disease are beyond the age of 65 years. Cardiovascular disease was responsible for 38% of the deaths of men and about 47% of women in 2008 [1].

During the last two decades a reduction of about 20% of the deaths due to cardiovascular diseases has been recorded. This reduction is attributed mainly to the new pharmaceutical and interventional modalities. Among these modalities, percutaneous coronary intervention (PCI) holds a leading position with a continuously increasing rate of use since the method was first used 30 years earlier. In 2006 about 290.00 coronary interventions were performed in Germany, a significant increase from the 180.000 interventions in 2000 and the 32.000 interventions in 1990 [2]. During this period the proportion of coronary angiographies followed by a PCI also increased and accounted for about 33% of all coronary angiographies in 2006 vs. 18% in 1990. On the other hand, the number of coronary artery bypass graft operations (CABG) has continuously declined during the last decade from 65.000 operations in 2000 to about 47.000 operations in 2008 [3].

Consequently, cardiovascular disease is the leading disease in health costs with 35 billion Euros spent on it in 2002 followed by the diseases of the gastrointestinal tract on which 31 billion Euros was spent in the same year. Ischemic heart disease alone costs 7 billion Euros per year [4].

1.1.2 Pathophysiology

Coronary artery disease (CAD) is identified by the presence of narrowing lesions within the coronary arterial tree. These stenotic lesions result from, and reflect, a series of alterations on the vascular wall in the chronic inflammatory process of atherosclerosis. Several risk factors, like age, male gender, obesity, and sedentary lifestyle, are thought to predispose an individual to atherosclerosis. The most important of the modifiable coronary risk factors appear to be hyperlipidemia, smoking, and diabetes. Atherosclerosis is a multifactorial disease that is characterized by interactions of different plasma lipoproteins, leukocytes, smooth muscle cells, and extracellular matrix compounds. The initial lesions of atherosclerosis, the fatty streak lesions, are often present in the aorta of children, the coronary arteries of adolescents, and other peripheral vessels of young adults without causing any clinical pathology at this stage. Through the accumulation of extracellular-matrix components, such as collagen from the vascular smooth muscle cells, the streak lesions are modified to atherosclerotic lesions. Later, inflammatory cells, such as monocytes and T cells, are recruited to atherosclerotic lesions and help to perpetuate a state of chronic inflammation. As the plaque grows, compensatory remodeling takes place so that the lumen is preserved while its overall diameter increases. Atherosclerosis appears to be clinically accessible primarily during middle age when a plaque ruptures, resulting in acute coronary syndrome, or encroaches on the lumen of the vessel causing obstructive coronary disease [5]. The narrowing in the coronary arteries results in an imbalance between oxygen supply and oxygen demand in the myocardium. The severity of the myocardial ischemia depends on the magnitude of the coronary artery disease, the number of coronary arteries with atherosclerotic lesions and the degree of the stenosis. Ischemic heart disease (IHD) is another term used to describe the clinical manifestations of atherosclerosis that is caused by a significantly reduced blood flow to a region of the heart. Ischemic heart disease, when symptomatic, appears in various forms from stable angina to acute coronary syndromes (ACS) with or without ST elevation (STE-ACS and NSTE-ACS, respectively). A STE-ACS usually leads to an ST elevation myocardial infarction (STEMI), whereas the non-STE-ACS is further qualified as non-ST elevation MI (NSTEMI) or unstable angina [6].

1.1.3 Clinical features of stable coronary disease

Patients who have a stable CAD typically present (more than 70%) angina. The other 30% of patients who have coronary artery disease, mainly older patients, diabetics and women, present only atypical symptoms. The classical symptom of angina is chest discomfort due to myocardial ischemia. This occurs as a specific myocardial oxygen requirement that cannot be met by a myocardial oxygen supply itself. This is the case in the presence of coronary artery disease where one or more coronary arteries are significant narrowed. However, angina may also be present in the absence of epicardial stenoses. In these cases, structural or functional disorders of the heart muscle and coronary arteries may compromise coronary blood flow relative to myocardial oxygen demand, thereby causing angina. For example, we refer to microvascular angina or syndrome X, hypertensive heart disease, ventricular cardiomyopathies or vasospastic angina. The discomfort caused by myocardial ischemia is usually located in the chest, arms, jaw, teeth or, neck (Buddenbrooks syndrome), between the shoulder blades, epigastrium and/or interscapular areas.

Patients use different terms to describe the angina, such as tightness, pressure, heaviness, burning, aching or penetration. In addition to chest discomfort, typical angina is often associated with a specific factor that is identified as the trigger of an ischemic event. Angina is high reproducible when this factor is present. In most of the cases, exertion is the trigger, although stress, cold or meals have also been associated with the appearance of angina. Relief of the symptoms occurs after rest or intake of nitroglycerine. In the majority of the cases, the duration of the symptoms is brief, usually less than 10 minutes. Angina may also be accompanied by shortness of breath and less specific symptoms, such as fatigue or faintness, nausea, burping or restlessness. Patients who have diabetes may have no symptoms (silent ischemia) or may present with exercise-induced dyspnea as an angina equivalent [7].

Some patients experience atypical angina, which consists only of two of the three main characteristics of typical angina: chest symptoms, presence of a triggering factor and relief due to rest or nitroglycerine.

The main dissociation of angina is between stable and unstable angina. With stable angina, the symptoms exist for a long time, and appear at the same level of exertion, with a stable frequency and intensity. Each episode lasts about 10 minutes. If, within a few days, the frequency or the duration of the episodes increases or the angina-threshold declines, an unstable angina is present. The possibility of a NSTE-ACS or STE-ACS/STEMI in patients with unstable angina is raised, particularly when symptoms have been unremitting for more than 20 minutes.

Other conditions, such as hypertrophic cardiomyopathy, hypertensive crisis, valvular heart disease or myocarditis, may be associated with typical symptoms of NSTE-ACS. Other conditions, such as Prinzmetal´s angina or pericarditis, may have a similar clinical and electrocardiographic feature with a STE-ACS [6].

1.1.4 Diagnostic tests

In addition to the history, physical examination and rest electrocardiography (ECG), several invasive and non-invasive tests are used to assess patients who have a suspected or known stable coronary artery disease. In addition to the patient history, different scores may be used for risk stratification of the patient (Framingham-score, PROCAM-Score) and the arrangement of further diagnostic or interventional procedures. An exercise ECG is generally conducted for most patients who have angina or an intermediate probability for coronary disease based on age, gender, and symptoms. When resting ECG abnormalities are present, the exercise ECG may be invaluable. In this case, or when an exercise ECG is contraindicated, a non-invasive imaging test is performed. Non-invasive stress imaging techniques have several advantages over conventional exercise ECG testing. These include superior diagnostic performance for the detection of obstructive coronary disease and the ability to quantify and localize areas of ischemia. These tests also provide useful diagnostic information for patients who have resting ECG abnormalities or are unable to exercise [7]. The most commonly used imaging tests are stress echocardiography and myocardial scintigraphy (SPECT-single photon emission computed tomography). Both tests can be performed in combination with exercise that provides a physiological reproduction of exercise--induced myocardial ischemia. If the exercise level is inadequate, or the patient is unable to exercise, a pharmacological stimulus with dobutamine or adenosine is usually applied. Stress echocardiography and stress scintigraphy generally provide similar accuracy in the detection of CAD, although perfusion imaging is slightly more sensitive (84%) than stress-echo (80%). On the other hand, stress-echocardiography is slightly more specific (86%) than scintigraphy (77%) [8]. Positron emission tomography (PET) is also used to assess myocardial blood flow with a high sensitivity and a better spatial resolution and more accurate attenuation correction than SPECT [9]. Over the last few years, the application of cardiac magnetic resonance (CMR) for the detection and prognosis of CAD has gained attention. High spatial resolution myocardial perfusion cardiac magnetic resonance CMR with adenosine has a sensitivity of 87-90% and a specificity of 83-85% compared to coronary angiography [10]. CMR also has a very high prognostic value. A normal adenosine CMR predicts a three-year event-free survival with an accuracy of 99.2% [11]. Recent data support the use of computed tomography coronary angiography (CTCA) for symptomatic patients who have suspected CAD. It has been shown that CTCA has a higher diagnostic accuracy than exercise ECG or SPECT in predicting CAD and, consequently, in referring patients for angiography [12]. Although non-invasive tests are increasingly used in the diagnosis of CAD, coronary angiography remains the gold standard in the investigation of patients who have CAD. It provides reliable anatomical information to identify the presence or absence of coronary lumen stenosis, to define therapeutic options and to determine prognosis [7]. In the presence of several coronary artery stenoses, or when a stenosis is suspected to cause ischemia under exertion, the fractional flow reserve (FFR), as calculated by coronary pressure measurement, is the invasive gold standard for assessing the hemodynamic significance of a stenosis. FFR reliably indicates whether a stenosis is responsible for an inducible ischemia and whether a percutaneous coronary intervention is appropriate.

1.1.5 Therapy for stable CAD

1.1.5.1 Secondary prevention

The most important action to reduce mortality and morbidity by CAD is to control the risk factors that cause the disease. The Framingham study identified the following major risk factors for coronary artery disease: age, gender, blood pressure, total and high-density cholesterol, smoking and glucose intolerance [13]. According to international guidelines, control of all the above modifiable risk factors is necessary for patients who have angina (class I recommendation) [14]. Control of blood pressure control under 140/90 mm Hg or 130/80 mm Hg for patients who have diabetes or chronic kidney disease is indicated. Furthermore, low density lipoprotein (LDL) should be less than 100 mg/dl, while a further intensification of the therapy towards an LDL target of 70 mg/dl is associated with a further reduction of mortality from CAD and the incidence of non-fatal cardiovascular events [15]. All patients should be encouraged to participate in 30 to 60 minutes of a moderate-intensity aerobic activity, such as brisk walking, during most days of the week. Cessation of smoking, control of body weight (body mass index (BMI) <25kg/m^2) and management of diabetes to achieve a near-normal HbA$_{1C}$ = 6,5-7% are also indicated as secondary preventive measures for stable CAD [14].

1.1.5.2 Medical treatment

Pharmacological treatment of patients who have coronary artery disease is recommended to improve the prognosis and reduce the ischemic symptoms. Antiplatelet therapy with aspirin is essential for all patients to prevent arterial thrombosis. The optimal antithrombotic dosage of aspirin is 75-150 mg/day. For patients who cannot take aspirin due to intolerance or allergic complications, an intake of 75mg/day of clopidogrel is recommended [7]. In addition to the antiplatelet therapy, treatment with statins should be also prescribed for all patients who have stable coronary artery disease [16]. The recommended dose of statin may vary, but the aim is to reduce the LDL-cholesterol to a level below 70 mg/dl [14]. If the high density lipoprotein (HDL) is low and the triglyceride levels remain high, other pharmaceutical substances may be added to statin to treat the severe dyslipidemia of the patient. The use of beta-blockers is generally recommended for all patients who have CAD and a myocardial infarction and as a first-line anti-angina therapy for all CAD patients who have angina. If there is heart failure after myocardial infarction, and if a beta-blocker is contraindicated or not tolerated by the patient, use of a calcium channel blocker is desirable [17]. All patients who have stable angina should be considered for angiotensin-converting enzyme inhibitors (ACE-inhibitors), particularly if a need for ACE-inhibition is indicated, such as by hypertension, heart failure, left ventricular (LV) systolic dysfunction, prior myocardial infarction (MI) with LV dysfunction or diabetes [7]. Others suggest the use of ACE inhibitors in combination with aspirin, statin and beta-blocker for all patients who have coronary disease, regardless of the left ventricular function [18]. The reduction of anginal symptoms is also essential for patients who have a stable CAD. In the case of anginal attacks, short-acting nitrates are used for the immediate relief of symptoms. For long-term control of angina, beta 1-blockers are recommended. If the symptoms are not controlled, it may be necessary to add a calcium-blocker or a long-acting nitrate. Other agents, such as potassium channel openers or sinus node inhibitors (such as ivabradine), may be used in addition to, or as an alternative to, the standard anti-anginal therapy if the patient remains symptomatic under different combinations of the standard therapy and various attempts at dose optimization [7].

1.1.5.3 Percutaneous coronary intervention (PCI) and coronary bypass surgery (CABG)

Revascularization procedures are recommended to improve prognosis and symptoms in patients who have stable angina. Based on the coronary artery anatomy, CABG is preferred to PCI if there is a significant stenosis of the left main artery or if the patient has a three-vessel disease. CABG for patients with multi-vessel disease is associated with a lower five-year mortality than percutaneous transluminal coronary angioplasty (PTCA) [19]. Outside the area of an acute coronary syndrome, where PCI reduces mortality and the incidence of myocardial infarction, PCI in patients who have stable CAD is mainly effective in relieving symptoms and improving the quality of life [20]. If the objective of revascularization is the relief of symptoms, then PCI is necessary for patients who have mild to moderate angina without any multi-vessel disease. Revascularization is not recommended for patients who have a single or two-vessel disease with mild symptoms or a borderline stenosis of 50-70% in a location other than the left main coronary artery [7]. However, other guidelines recommend PCI as a valuable initial revascularization procedure for all patients who have stable CAD and large objective ischemia [21]. The current data support benefits of PCI only in the symptoms and quality of life. The COURAGE trial demonstrated that, even for patients who have significant artery disease, adding PCI to the medical treatment does not decrease the rate of deaths, myocardial infarctions or hospitalization for acute coronary syndromes [22]. However, PCI has proved more effective in reducing episodes of angina and the need for revascularization. In accordance with this, a sub-study of the COURAGE trial demonstrated that a combination of PCI and optimal medical therapy (OMT) leads to a significant reduction of the inducible ischemia, when compared to OMT alone, particularly for patients who have severe ischemia at the baseline (>10% of myocardium) [23]. For patients who are unsuitable for further revascularization procedures (PCI or CABG) and who remain symptomatic, alternative therapeutic options for relief of symptoms are available. These include neurostimulation (transcutaneous electrical nerve stimulation and spinal cord stimulation), transmyocardial or percutaneous laser revascularization and external counterpulsation therapy [24].

1.2 Arteriogenesis

1.2.1 Terminology of vascular growth

The term neovascularization refers to the following three mechanisms of vascular growth that take place under physiological and pathological conditions:

- Vasculogenesis is a mechanism that is specific to the development of the circulatory system and new vessels during embryogenesis. Precursors cells called angioblasts differentiate to hematopoietic cells and to endothelial cells, which form the primary blood vessels [25]. Vasculogenesis may also occur in adults under pathological conditions (e.g., tumor progression). However, its importance as a therapeutic goal is limited as it leads only to an immature, poorly functional vasculature.

- Angiogenesis is defined as the sprouting of capillaries from pre-existing vessels resulting in new capillary networks [25]. This process is important for wound healing in granulation tissue. However, at the same time, it is part of pathological conditions like diabetic retinopathy and vascularization of tumors. The new capillary networks consist of endothelial cell tubes that lack additional wall structures, such as smooth muscle cells or adventitia, which stabilize the structures and cells. The absence of muscle cells prevents the capillaries from filling perfusion needs by dilation or constriction as the larger vessels (arterioles) do. The main triggers of angiogenesis are tissue hypoxia and inflammation. After occlusion of an artery, angiogenesis takes place in the distal ischemic tissue far from the site of occlusion [26]. The new capillaries could only compensate for the tissue hypoxia and supply the tissue with oxygen if an open feeding artery were available [27]. Furthermore, the perfusion pressure in the developed capillaries is very low and not sufficient enough to ensure an adequate oxygenation of the tissues. The absence of a stable arterial wall structure makes also the capillaries prone to rupture and vulnerable to external pressures. The perfusion pressure in the capillaries may be further diminished in the case of increased tissue pressure, a condition that is often encountered due to increased left ventricular diastolic pressure [28]. Thus, development of new capillaries is rather inadequate as compensation for the deficit in perfusion due to artery occlusion, especially in the myocardium.

- The third mechanism of neovascularization called arteriogenesis refers to the development of collateral arteries from pre-existing arteries / arterioles. The term arteriogenesis was proposed to distinguish this process from angiogenesis. Both processes seek to compensate for hypo- perfusion, but differ in many aspects. The main characteristics of angiogenesis and arteriogenesis are summarized in Figure 1-1. Common characteristics include the role of growth factors and leukocyte populations.

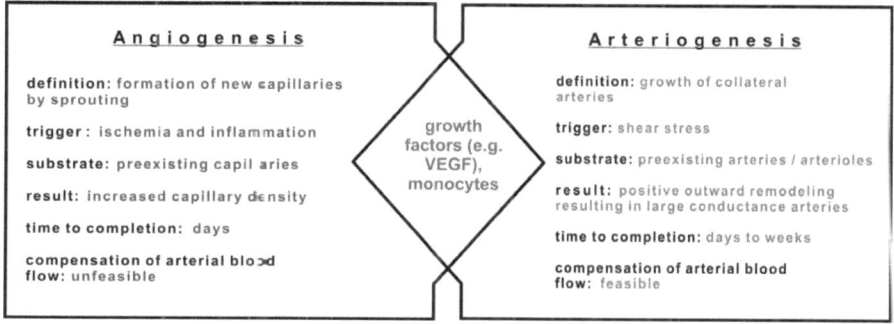

Figure 1-1: *Main characteristics of arteriogenesis and angiogenesis [29]*

1.2.2 Collateral artery growth and the role of shear stress

Arteriogenesis occurs in response to occlusion or stenosis of an artery. Substrates of arteriogenesis are pre-existing collaterals that can grow up to 25 times their original size and become small arteries. These small arterioles are part of a network that interconnect perfusion territories of arterial sub branches [30]. In a normal human heart there are numerous superficial (epicardial) or deep (transeptal or subendocardial) anastomoses (Figure 1-2A).

The deep anastomoses are generally larger in diameter (100-200µm) and more numerous than the superficial arterioles [31]. In ischemic hearts, the enlarged collateral vessels derive from these anastomoses (Figure 1-2B).

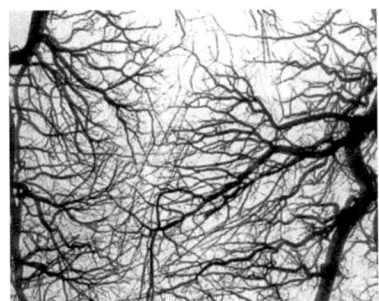 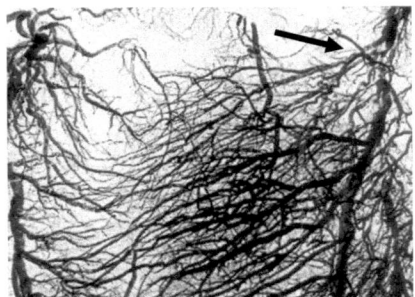

Figure 1-2A: *Anastomoses in a normal heart.*   Figure 1-2B: *Collateral arteries after occlusion of the LAD (arrow)*

(from [32]:Chapter 16, page 303,Figures 4-5 by permission of Springer Science and Business Media)

The major stimulus for the enlargement of the pre-existing arterioles is the presence of a significant arterial stenosis or occlusion. In this case, a pressure gradient develops between the proximal and distal parts of the narrowed or occluded artery. This pressure drop leads to an increase of the blood flow through the interconnecting network. As the pressure gradient increases in proportion to the severity of the stenosis, the blood flow from the donor artery to the ischemic territory is augmented. The increased blood flow results in an increase of the fluid shear stress and the wall tension in the growing arteries, which are the major forces that trigger the process of arteriogenesis [30]. The fluid shear stress (τ) is proportional to the blood flow (Q) and the blood viscosity (η) and inversely related to the radius (R) of the vessel:

$$\text{Equation 1-1:} \quad \tau = \frac{4\eta Q}{R^3 \pi}$$

The response of the collateral arteries to the increased blood flow is not only a passive dilatation, but also an active structural enlargement [33, 34]. The increased blood flow that results in enhanced endothelial shear stress within these arteriolar/arterial anastomoses activates the endothelium [(e.g., by increased transcription of the transient receptor potential action channel, subfamily V, member 4 (Trpv4)]. This receptor senses enhanced shear levels and converts them to the Ca^{2+} signal, which in turn, participates in regulation of cell volume, endothelial permeability and initial vascular dilatation [35]. Shear stress and wall stretch activate the vascular endothelium and the vascular muscle cells to express the monocyte chemoattractant protein (MCP-1). The MCP-1 is regarded as a critical determinant for the process of arteriogenesis [36]. Attracted by the MCP-1, circulating monocytes adhere to and invade the endothelium. Growth factors released from macrophages induce a proliferation of endothelial and smooth muscle cells (SMCs). The monocytes express proteases like matrix-metalloproteinases, which degrade the vessel wall to permit the migration of SMCs [37]. The complex interplay of circulating cells, growth factors, different proteins and structural changes result in functional arteries. The conductance of the collateral arteries is much greater than that of the pre-existing arterioles from which they derived. These arterioles/collateral arteries can compensate, in part at least, for the reduced blood flow caused by the narrowing or occlusion of the main feeding artery. In a rabbit hind limb model of chronic occlusion of the femoral artery, collateral arteries can restore the perfusion distal to the occlusion up to ≈35% of the normal conductance. However, the increase in the diameter of the arterioles as a response to the occlusion of the feeding arteries leads to a normalization of the initial increased shear stress. As long as shear stress is the trigger of arteriogenesis, its early normalization due to an increase in the vessel's diameter results in a premature halt to the arteriogenic process. Eitenmueller et al [38] showed that if the shear stress remains at an increased level throughout arteriogenesis (e.g., with an arterio-venous shunt), collateral vessels may completely restore the conductance of the occluded artery. In addition to the time-course of shear stress, the level of fluid shear stress plays an important role in collateral growth.

In humans, shear stress may be increased by exercise training and/or the presence of a significant stenosis. It has been suggested that the severity of the stenosis is the only independent variable that is related to collateral growth in patients who have CAD [39]. The increase in the grade of a stenosis leads to an increased pressure gradient to the interconnecting collateral channels. This translates to an elevated blood flow and shear stress resulting in arteriogenesis [40].

1.2.3 The protective role of coronary collateral circulation

The beneficial effects of the coronary collateral circulation have been demonstrated in patients who have chronic coronary disease and acute myocardial infarction. The severity of an infarction depends on the time between onset of the infarction and revascularization and the presence of collateral vessels [41]. Though that the presence of collaterals at the time of infarction is not directly related to the size of the infarction, lower rates of formation of left ventricular aneurysms occur in the presence of collateral arteries. It has been hypothesized that, due to collateral arteries, "islands" of viable myocardium are maintained amidst the infarction's area, thereby enforcing its tensile strength, preventing aneurysm formation and maintaining the ventricular function [42, 43]. The presence of collateral arteries is also related to lower rates of non-fatal cardiac events [44]. Hansen et al [45] showed that patients with angiographically well developed collaterals (based on Bruschke's classification [46]) had a 10-year survival rate that was superior to that of patients who are without collateral arteries and that this benefit was related to lower rates of heart failure. These data were recently verified using the pressure-derived collateral flow index by Meier et al [47]. The investigators showed that a low CFIp (< 0.25) is independently associated with increased mortality of patients who have stable coronary disease in a 10-year follow-up. A CFIp<0.25 is predictive of more future major cardiac events than well developed collaterals that are characterized by a CFIp>0.25 [48]. An important issue concerning collateral growth is the dependence of collateral development on the time taken for the arterial obstruction to develop. A slow progression of the disease, often related to repeated angina episodes, may be associated with a better collateral network [49]. Whether these angina episodes (known as "walking through angina") are a phenomenon of collateral recruitment, ischemic preconditioning, or both, remains unclear [50, 51]. In summary, not only the acute outcome, but also the long-term survival following a myocardial infarction depends on the extent of collateral circulation [52].

1.2.4 Assessment of cardiac collateral arteries

1.2.4.1 Non-invasive methods

The current non-invasive imaging techniques provide useful data for the perfusion territory supplied by collateral arteries, but at present lack the accuracy of the invasive gold standards. Positron emission tomography is useful for quantification of collateral-dependent myocardium, but it cannot be used as a routine method for collateral assessment. Myocardial contrast echocardiography is another potential method for assessing collateral supply. An important weakness of these non-invasive methods is that they can be performed only if the coronary status is already known by coronary angiography. The angiography is necessary to disclose the site of a coronary occlusion or severe stenosis and consequently permit the non-invasive estimation of the area provided with collateral blood flow [53]

1.2.4.2 Angiographic methods

Coronary angiography is one of the most frequent applied methods for visual assessment of coronary collateral circulation. However, for a reliable assessment of collateral arteries, a model of coronary occlusion must be present - either the natural occlusion model (chronic total occlusion) or an artificial coronary occlusion model with a brief blocking of the vessel by an angioplasty balloon catheter [54]. Rentrop's classification (often used with modifications) is the most commonly used test to assess visible and recruitable collaterals. During natural or artificial occlusion of the culprit artery, dye is injected into the contralateral artery. The following score describes the filling of the epicardial artery with contrast dye by collaterals: 0 = no visible collateral channel filling; 1 = filling of side branches of the occluded artery without visualization of the epicardial segment; 2 = partial filling of the epicardial segment by collateral channels; 3 = complete filling of the epicardial segment of the culprit artery [55]. If the culprit lesion is not occluded, but only narrowed, a double artery approach (e.g. via both femoral arteries) is required for the simultaneously brief occlusion and dye injection, a major limitation of the method.

Rockstroh and colleagues [56] reported on an another quantitative angiographic analysis of the collateral diameter and underscored the relevance of it for the collateral function. For this analysis, four types of collaterals are distinguished: septal (SE), atrial (AT), branch-branch in ventricular free walls (BR), and bridging across lesions (BL). Three different frames of a collateral artery and three different points on the collateral artery are used. From these images, nine different measurements are made. The average of these values constitutes the collateral artery diameter [56].

Using the above anatomical classification of the collaterals, Werner et al. suggested another classification (three-grade system) for the connecting collaterals (CC): CC 0, no continuous connection between donor and recipient artery; CC 1, a continuous, threadlike connection; and CC 2, a continuous, small side branch-like size of the collateral throughout its course. The size is estimated by using an electronic caliper on enlarged still images: CC1 collaterals diameter ≤0.3 mm and CC2 ≥0.4 mm) [57]. The authors showed that this grading system correlates to the invasive determinants of the collateral hemodynamics, such as the collateral resistance index (Rcoll). However, the angiographic methods, although widely used, are generally limited in accuracy, as the visible assessment of the collaterals is subject to intra- and inter- observer error and only spontaneous visible collaterals are detected [58].

1.2.4.3 Intracoronary functional measurements

At present, the most valuable method for assessing coronary collateral artery function is based on intracoronary pressure and flow measurements. Perfusion pressure and flow velocity obtained distally to occluded arteries are considered to derive from the collateral vessels [54]. By using a guidewire with pressure or Doppler-sensors, the functional status of the collateral circulation can be evaluated during coronary angiography. A prerequisite for the calculation of the conductance of the collateral arteries is the transient creation of an artificial occlusion of the diseased coronary artery with a PCI-balloon. By measuring simultaneously the aortic and the intracoronary pressure or velocity distally to the occlusion, a pressure-derived or velocity-derived collateral flow index (CFI) is calculated [59]. The CFI index expresses the amount of collateral flow to the region of interest distally to the occlusion as a fraction of the normal flow, if the vessel was patent.

The collateral flow pressure-derived index (CFIp) is calculated by the aortic pressure (Pa), the intracoronary pressure under balloon inflation (wedge pressure-Pw) and the central venous pressure (Pv):

$$\text{Equation 1-2: } CFIp = \frac{Pw - Pv}{Pa - Pv}$$

Pa, Pw, Pv (all in mm of Hg) are mean pressure values that are registered at the end of an one-minute coronary occlusion, as explained in Chapter 3.4.2 [60]. The Pv, measured in the right atrium, must be subtracted from both the aortic and distal pressures in order to obtain an accurate value for the CFIp index [61]. The pressure-derived collateral index is validated by scintigraphy for the semi-quantification of the collateral flow [62]. In the presence of an epicardial stenosis, a pressure derived collateral index greater than 0.30 (no units) suggests a collateral flow that is sufficient to prevent myocardial ischemia during PCI [59] and is related to a low rate of ischemic events after PCI of the vessel [61]. Data from large databases suggest that a cut-off value of 0.25 differentiates patients with well (CFIp>0.25) or poorly (CFIp<0.25) developed collaterals [47].

An analogue to CFIp, the velocity-derived collateral flow index (CFIv) expresses collateral flow as a fraction of the flow provided by the normally patent artery. For its calculation, a guide wire with a Doppler-sensor is used. CFIv is calculated by measuring the coronary flow velocity distally to an occlusion (Voccl) and the coronary flow velocity during vessel patency (Vpat):

$$\text{Equation 1-3: } CFIv = \frac{Voccl}{Vpat}$$

Collateral flow velocity and pressure indices show good correlation with possibly greater sensitivity of the flow index at very low collateral flow index values [59, 63]. However, calculation of both indices has limitations. For accurate CFIv measurements, the location of the Doppler wire must be exactly the same during occlusion and vessel patency. Other causes of overestimation of the CFIv are signal artifacts due to wall movements. Furthermore, flow velocity during occlusion (Voccl) and flow velocity during patency of the vessel (Vpat) are not evaluated simultaneously and therefore are subject to hemodynamic (e.g., heart rate, aortic pressure) alterations. Overestimation of the CFIp may occur if the left ventricular end-diastolic pressure is increased (LVEDP>18mmHg) [64]. For reliable estimation of both indices, a constant coronary artery diameter, maintained by injection of nitroglycerine is important [65]. When pressure and flow measurements are performed successively, the estimation of indices of the collateral resistance is possible. Collateral resistance (Rcoll) consists of the collateral microvascular resistance and the resistance of the donor artery. Rcoll is inversely related to the extent of functional collateralization and is therefore used as an additional index of collateral artery status [66].

1.2.5 Clinical trials for the stimulation of arteriogenesis

The present data regarding the therapeutic induction of arteriogenesis by administration of pharmaceutical agents or other interventions, such as exercise, are limited. In a placebo-controlled study, Seiler et al [67] showed that CAD patients who received granulocyte-macrophage colony-stimulating factor (GM-CSF) had a significant increase in the CFIp compared to those who received placebo therapy. However, in the last mentioned trial, a high interindividual response to therapy was observed. Furthermore, there are serious concerns about the safety of colony-stimulating factors in patients who have CAD [68]. Other investigators have used several growth factors, primarily from the family of FGF (fibroblast growth factor) and VEGF (vascular endothelial growth factor) to promote angiogenesis, arteriogenesis or both. The VIVA trial [69] did not show any benefit for patients who received recombinant human vascular endothelial growth factor protein (rhVEGF) in comparison to the placebo group.

Beyond growth factors, physical activity is also associated with the presence of sufficient collateral arteries [70]. In 23 patients who had ischemic heart disease, Belardinelli et al. [71] showed a significant improvement of the collateral arteries in response to eight weeks of endurance training, whereas, in another study, there was no angiographic improvement of collaterals after one year of training [72]. Zbinden et al. [73] suggested that even normal coronary arteries of CAD patients can be supplied with increased collateral flow in response to exercise, suggesting that, even in the absence of ischemia, collateral artery growth take place from pre-existing collaterals. The controversy surrounding the data above may be explained by the different methods used to assess the formation of collaterals. Thus, the supposed arteriogenic effect of exercise continues to have not been clearly demonstrated in large clinical trials.

1.3 External Counterpulsation

1.3.1 Introduction

The term external counterpulsation refers to a non-invasive device that is used to achieve a diastolic augmentation analogue to the intra-aortic balloon counterpulsation. External counterpulsation was initially developed to help patients with acute myocardial infarction and heart failure as a non-invasive alternative technique to the intra-aortic balloon (IABP) [74-76]. The first experiments and clinical trials with external counterpulsation took place about 40 years ago in an investigation of the acute hemodynamic effects on the left ventricular workload and the coronary perfusion [77-79]. However, the first hydraulic counterpulsation device proved to be less effective than IABP for the treatment of cardiogenic shock [80]. An alternative non-invasive counterpulsation device that was based on air-filled cuffs came into use in the late 1970s [81]. The currently used counterpulsation systems are based on the latter. Despite the different commercial names of the available devices of external counterpulsation (enhanced external counterpulsation [EECP], increased external counterpulsation {IECP}, sequential external counterpulsation [SECP]), the physiologic principles of the devices are the same. To avoid misunderstandings, only the term external counterpulsation (ECP) will be used in this manuscript.

ECP is indicated in the treatment of the refractory angina pectoris today as suggested by the guidelines (recommendation class IIb [7]). Other approved indications for use include unstable angina, congestive heart failure, acute myocardial infarction and cardiogenic shock [82]. The clinical benefits for patients with CAD include diminution of anginal symptoms, reduced uptake of nitroglycerine, increase in exercise tolerance and improvement in the quality of life [83]. Three of four patients with refractory angina experience an improvement in at least one class in the classification of the Canadian Cardiovascular Society of Cardiology (CCS) and 38% of them experience improvements in at least two classes immediately following the therapy. The benefits for most of the patients can be maintained for up to three years after completion of the therapy [84]. The exercise capacity of the majority of patients [85-87] is also improved. Recent studies have demonstrated the safety and effectiveness of the method for patients with mild to moderate heart failure. Exercise tolerance and functional class in the New York Heart Association (NYHA) classification were also improved following the therapy [88]. A retrospective analysis of patients who have refractory angina and underwent ECP revealed a significant reduction of systolic pressure [89]. The therapy may also be effective for other conditions, such as hepatorenal syndrome [90], restless leg syndrome [91], erectile dysfunction [92], tinnitus [93] and, as has been shown recently, ischemic stroke [94].

1.3.2 Technique of ECP

Three pairs of cuffs are wrapped around the calves and lower and upper thighs to augment blood flow. The cuffs are inflated from distal to proximal during early diastole and are deflated at the onset of systole (Figure 1-3). This mechanism results in augmented diastolic pressure (diastolic augmentation) and increased venous return during inflation. Due to the rapid deflation at the onset of systole, the peripheral vascular resistance is lowered (systolic unloading).

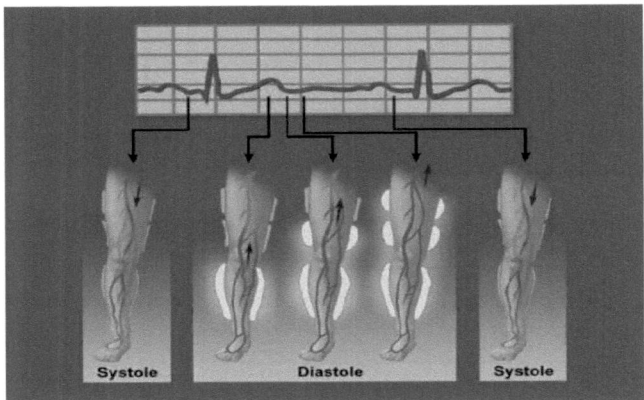

Figure 1-3: *Principle of enhanced external counterpulsation (from www.mayoclinic.org, Copyright 2009 Mayo Foundation for Medical Education and Research)*

The synchronization of the cuff compressions with the cardiac cycle takes place automatically through ECG. The hemodynamic impact of the ECP device is monitored in real-time with finger plethysmography. During inflation-deflation, finger plethysmography displays the diastolic and systolic alterations of the blood volume respectively. These changes in the blood volume on the finger's tip reflect alterations of the vascular bed due to the ECP (Figure 1-4).

Whereas the principal operation of ECP is ECG-triggered and automatic, the operator can optimize the hemodynamic effect by modifying the times of inflation and deflation of the cuffs. For example, a prolongation of the inflation time results in a longer compression of the cuffs. These adjustments of times are based on the achieved diastolic and systolic curves that are depicted continuously on the device's monitor. From these curves, the D/S ratio is calculated automatically as: *D/S ratio= diastolic augmentation amplitude / systolic augmentation amplitude*. An increase in the ratio reflects reduced peripheral vascular resistance and an improved endothelial function. Previous trials have shown that an increase in the ratio during the treatment period is related to the reduction in angina class and an improved outcome of the therapy [95, 96]. However, other trials suggest that the therapy is effective independently of an improvement of the ratio, supporting the belief that a more complex action mechanism, as described below, is behind the clinical effect of ECP [97]. A maximal hemodynamic effect is achieved by an index of 1.5 or greater [98].

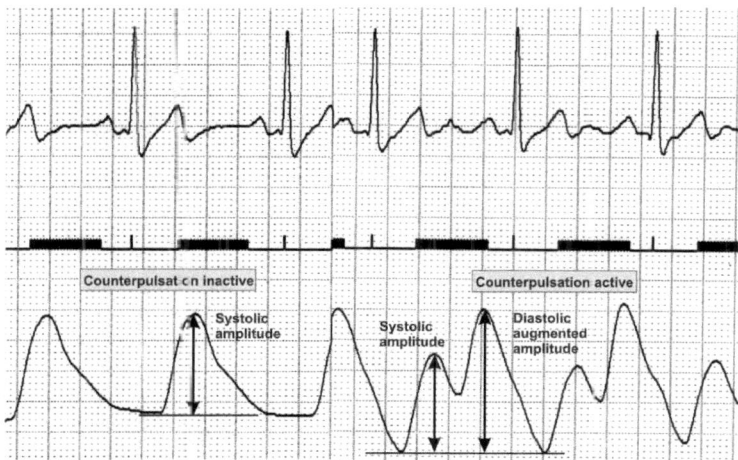

Figure 1.4: *Finger plethysmography curves as transmitted by the counterpulsation machine. Before activation of ECP only a systolic wave can be seen. Right, after activation of ECP a second diastolic wave is produced. The D/S ratio is calculated from these amplitudes.*

A typical course of EECP includes 35 outpatient treatments administered as 1-hour daily sessions over seven weeks. This standard duration of counterpulsation treatment is based on empirical data derived from studies in China and has been proposed as the optimal course based on data from the international EECP® Patient Registry [99].

1.3.3 Mechanism of the action and review of the literature

Although the technical principle of external counterpulsation is simple, the physiological response, especially that of hemodynamic effects, is complex and the mechanisms of action are only partially elucidated. Three main hypotheses have been accepted so far, but are still under investigation: i.) adaptive proliferation of coronary collateral arteries (arteriogenesis), ii) improvement of the endothelial function and decrease of peripheral resistance, iii) improvement of the left ventricular function. The links among these hypotheses are presented in Figure 1-5.

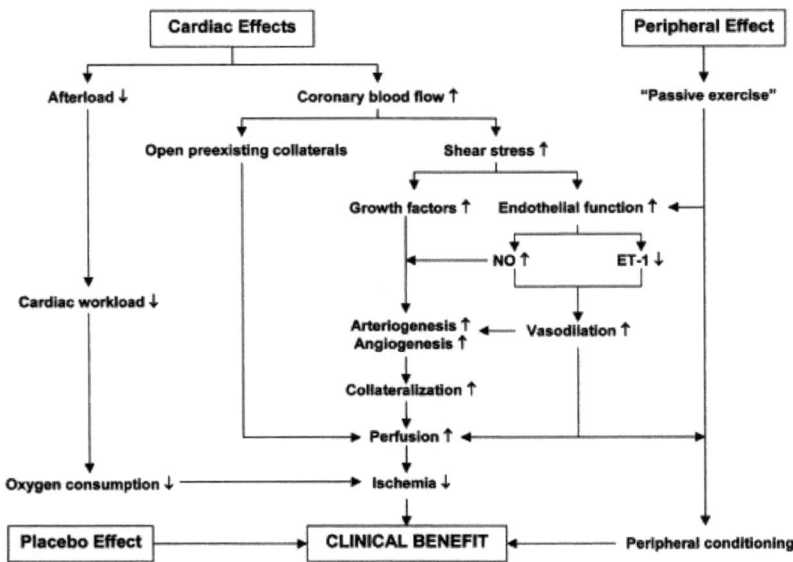

Figure 1-5: *Mechanism of the action of external counterpulsation (reprinted from [100] with permission from Elsevier)*

The first two hypotheses share a biomechanical effect of ECP - the increase in shear stress. Michaels and colleagues investigated the acute effect of ECP on cardiac function and circulation by intracoronary pressure measurements and intracoronary Doppler flow. They showed that intracoronary peak diastolic pressure was increased by 93% during ECP, while peak systolic pressure was reduced by 15%. The peak diastolic coronary flow velocity was increased by 109%, suggesting an improvement in coronary blood velocity [101]. In another study, the blood flow in the brachial artery was increased, although the diameter of the artery remained unchanged [102]. According to the latter data and Equation 1-1, it is assumed that the shear stress in the arterial system is increased during ECP. Increased levels of shear stress are crucial for the maintenance and improvement of endothelial function, as well as for arteriogenesis [103, 104]. The improved endothelial function leads to improved vasodilatation, which forms a crucial regulatory mechanism of the myocardial blood flow. In addition, the vasodilatation is important for the supply of blood to the collateral arteries during arteriogenesis [105]. The hypotheses of arteriogenesis and endothelial function are discussed below in detail.

1.3.3.1 ECP and Collateral Arteries

The hypothesis of arteriogenesis as a mechanism of action of counterpulsation goes back to the 1970s. Jacobey and Rosenzweig examined post mortem angiograms of dogs that were initially submitted to an acute or chronic myocardial infarction and consequently treated with counterpulsation therapy. The angiograms showed enhanced epicardial and sub-endocardial collateralization and reduced size of infarction in dogs that were treated with counterpulsation in comparison to control dogs [106, 107]. In a recent study, canines with myocardial ischemia were treated with an external counterpulsation model that was similar to that which is currently used in humans. The animals were submitted to occlusion of a coronary artery before being randomized in the active ECP group or control group. After six weeks of counterpulsation, the perfusion defects in the initial ischemic infarcted areas were attenuated in the active group [108]. The improvement of the perfusion only in the ischemic areas suggests an angiogenic effect of the method. However, no data about perfusion changes in the myocardial areas near the ischemic regions were presented.

Several studies have investigated the effect of ECP on myocardial perfusion in humans. However, the data is controversial. Masuda et al [109] studied prospectively 11 patients with at least one coronary stenosis (> 90%) before and after treatment with ECP. Myocardial perfusion, assessed by dipyrimadole ^{13}N-ammonia positron emission tomography (PET), increased after ECP, suggesting an arteriogenic effect of the therapy [109]. Improved myocardial perfusion by myocardial scintigraphy and reduction of wall abnormalities assessed by stress-echocardiography are shown in many clinical trials. Two other studies showed no effect of ECP on myocardial perfusion, despite a clinical improvement of the patients accompanied by reduced peripheral resistances and decreased heart rate response to exercise [85, 110]. The authors attributed it to a "training effect." Other investigators assessed the impact of ECP on collateral arteries and myocardial perfusion invasively with angiographically scoring (Rentrop score) and non- invasively with SPECT [86]. Both endpoints were assessed before and after ECP in patients who had at least one residual coronary stenosis. The reduction of the perfusion defects in SPECT was not accompanied by a significant increase of the Rentrop score, but was related to a reduction of the left ventricular end-diastolic pressure (LVEDP) [86]. However, the visual principle of the Rentrop score does not allow the detection of collateral < 1mm and is subject to intra- and interobserver errors [58].

A summary of all trials that assess the effect of ECP on myocardial perfusion is presented in Table 1-1. Eight of eleven studies demonstrated that, after ECP, the reduced myocardial ischemia is correlated with an improvement of the anginal symptoms, thereby suggesting recruitment and proliferation of collaterals as the most probable mechanism. The growth of collateral arteries bypassing the stenosis or occlusion results in an improvement of regional perfusion at rest. Under exertion or during a stress-test, the blood flow by collaterals may further increase as recruitment of collaterals occurs under myocardial ischemia. This increased perfusion may alleviate the patient's anginal symptoms and be detected as an improved perfusion in scans.

1.3.3.2 ECP and Endothelial Dysfunction

The hypothesis of improvement of the endothelial function is already supported by clinical and experimental data. It is not only the increased shear stress, but also the increased number of arterial pulsations per cardiac cycle during the counterpulsation therapy that exerts beneficial effects on the endothelium [111]. During the therapy a second pulsation occurs during diastole for every heart beat. By performing functional tests for the assessment of the peripheral endothelial function, such as brachial artery flow-mediated dilation (FMD) or reactive hyperemia-peripheral arterial tonometry (RH-PAT), an improvement of the endothelial function in response to ECP has been shown [112, 113]. Circulating levels of important mediators of the endothelial function (cGMP and nitric oxide) are also elevated after ECP, suggesting a positive effect of the therapy on the endothelial function [114, 115]. Recently, it was reported that ECP reduces the circulating levels of inflammatory cytokines. Casey and colleagues demonstrated a reduction of the levels of the tumor necrosis factor-α (TNF-α), monocyte chemoattractant protein-1 (MCP-1) and vascular adhesion molecule -1 (VSCM-1) after ECP. Furthermore, stabilization of the endothelium, which also occurs after exercise training, was demonstrated in hyperocholsterolemic pigs in response to ECP [116].

Other investigators discovered that ECP reduces arterial stiffness, implicating a peripheral vasodilatation and decrease of the peripheral resistances due mostly to improved endothelial function [117]. An improvement of the arterial stiffness could have a direct effect on coronary perfusion. It is known that an increased artery stiffness attenuates coronary blood flow due to an increased left ventricular workload and a reduced coronary artery diastolic filling [118].

Table 1-1: *Clinical trials assessing the effect of ECP on myocardial ischemia by imaging stress tests*

Study (Ref. #)	N	Population / Design	Test(s) used	Results
[119]	18	Stable CAD, prospective trial	Treadmill thallium - 201 SPECT for the same exercise duration	Reduction of perfusion defects in 14 patients (78%, $p<0.01^*$)
[120]	50	Chronic stable angina, angiographic CAD (>70% stenosis in a major vessel), retrospective trial	Exercise radionuclide test at the same workload	i. Improvement of perfusion imaging ($p<0.001^*$), ii. inverse relation between CAD severity and therapeutic benefit ($p<0.01^*$)
[121]	60	2 groups of patients: Group A: unbypassed patients with 1-, 2- or 3- vessel disease. Group B: patients with prior CABG and residual 1-, 2- or 3 vessel disease, prospective trial	Treadmill radionuclide test at the same workload	i. Comparable effectiveness in patients of both groups with 1- or 2- vessel disease (88% in group A vs 80% in group B, p=NS) ii. improvement of 80% in group B vs 22% in A, p<0.05 (patients with 3-vessel disease)
[86]	12	Stable patients with stenotic lesions >75% in at least one major coronary artery, prospective trial	i. exercise thallium -201 SPECT, ii. coronary angiography with Rentrop score	i. Decrease of region with perfusion defects from 35% to 21% ($p<0.01^*$) after ECP ii. Rentrop score without significant change
[109]	11	Stable patients with >90% stenosis in at least one major coronary artery, prospective trial	Dipyridamole ^{13}N-ammonia positron emission tomography (PET)	i. Increase of the overall myocardial perfusion at rest ($p<0.05^*$) ii. increase of the dypiridamole myocardial perfusion only in the regions of CAD ($p<0.05^*$)
[122]	175	Patients with stable CAD. International seven-center study (the follow –up test was performed within 6 months after completion of the therapy)	Treadmill technetium - 99m sestamibi or thallium -201 SPECT to the same levels of exercise (4 centers or to the maximal workload after EECP (3 centers)	i. 83% improvement in perfusions defects of patients undergoing the test to the same level ii. 54% improvement in patients with maximal test post-ECP iii. higher improvement in patients with history of angioplasty vs patients with no history of revascularization (p<0.025)
[87]	25	Presence of stenosis >70% in one or more major coronary artery or a history of CABG. Prospective, two-center study.	Symptom-limited maximal technetium 99m sestamibi SPECT	64% of the patients had improved nuclear scores after EECP (from 16.36 to 14.12, $p<0.05^*$)
[123]	23	Stable refractory angina pectoris, prospective trial	Dobutamine stress echocardiography	Improvement ≥2 grades in wall motion scores in 43% of patients. Average change 5.3±3.8 vs -0.6±3.0 in the 57% with no improvement (p<0.007)
[124]	25	Refractory angina and at least one non-revascularisable stenosis, prospective trial	Dobutamine stress echocardiography	36% of patients with improvement of the ischemia (NS)
[85]	37	Severe angina (CCS III-IV) and positive ischemic test, prospective multi-center trial	Symptom-limited technetium 99m sestamibi SPECT	No improvement of the myocardial perfusion
[110]	11	Stable angina, angiographic CAD (>70% stenosis in a major vessel), prospective trial	Dipyridamole ^{13}N-ammonia PET	No improvement of the myocardial perfusion in the normal or ischemic areas

* compared to baseline, NS= not statistical significant

However, other researchers could not confirm a positive effect of counterpulsation on arterial stiffness despite an improvement of exercise capacity in a treadmill test [125]. Furthermore, most of the exercise tests within past ECP trials were performed at the same level of exercise (same double product) before and after ECP. In this case, reduced myocardial oxygen demand due to a peripheral training effect and lower peripheral vascular resistance could also explain the attenuation of perfusion defects and the relief of the patients' symptoms.

Changes in the cardiac endothelial function may also be detected in the imaging test as perfusion changes at rest or under exercise. It is therefore obvious that both improvement of the endothelial function or the collateral growth after ECP could be detected as improved myocardial perfusion in the imaging tests of the studies mentioned in the previous chapter. This fact does not exclude that both mechanisms of action may contribute in parallel or synergistically to the effects of ECP. In the majority of the ECP trials performed to date physical exercise tests (e.g., treadmill SPECT), but no pharmacologic tests, were used to evaluate the effect of ECP on myocardial blood flow. By using these methods one cannot exclude a possible contribution of the coronary endothelium to the coronary blood flow. It is known that an impaired coronary endothelium may partly contribute to the perfusion defects demonstrated by SPECT [126] or vice versa (i.e., that the improvement of the myocardial ischemia after ECP may be partly attributed to improved coronary endothelial function).

As long as ECP exerts systemic effects on the vasculature, it is reasonable to hypothesize that the coronary endothelium is also improved following the therapy. Indeed, patients who suffer from microvascular angina that was attributed to Syndrome X were treated successfully with ECP. After the therapy, clinical improvement and a reduction of regional ischemia in imaging tests were demonstrated [127, 128]. These data may support a direct improvement of the coronary endothelial function and a consequent increase of the myocardial blood flow after ECP. Unfortunately, an assessment of the endothelium-dependent coronary vasodilatation by injecting acetylcholine before and after ECP has not been conducted to date.

All theses data support the hypothesis that ECP improves the endothelial function and reduces peripheral resistance.

1.3.3.3 Further mechanisms / hypotheses of action of ECP

As mentioned above, the reduction of perfusion defects in SPECT was associated by Urano and Colleagues [86] to a reduction of the left ventricular end-diastolic pressure (LVEDP) [86]. Such an improvement of the left ventricular function has also been related to a significant reduction of the atrial natriuretic peptide (ANP) and brain natriuretic peptide (BNP) in response to a course of ECP [109]. The reduced myocardial oxygen demand and/or the improved coronary artery filling due to the reduced diastolic pressure could also explain the attenuation of myocardial perfusion defects [86]. Other investigators demonstrated that a marker of the left ventricular filling, the lung-heart ratio was reduced after ECP [129]. The decrease of the lung/heart ratio indicates a decrease in the LVEDP and left ventricular end diastolic volume [130].

In an echocardiographic trial, the left ventricular end-diastolic volume decreased after therapy and the left ventricular ejection fraction (LVEF), when it was abnormal at baseline, increased after ECP [131]. However, in a recently published study, no improvement of any index of the left ventricular systolic and diastolic function was detected by echocardiography [132]. So, the effect of ECP on the function of the left ventricle must be studied in larger trials before a satisfactory conclusion can be drawn.

Another hypothesis of the mechanism of action suggested that the latter is an improvement of the autonomic regulation of coronary blood flow in response to ECP. The investigators assumed that an improvement of the function of the carotid baroreceptors due to the augmented diastolic aortic pressure could further improve the balance of the coronary autonomic tone. This could result in a decrease of the sympathetic tone and an improvement of coronary vasodilatation and coronary flow. However, the latter hypothesis could not be verified in a clinical trial [133] that assessed the heart rate variability pre and post EECP as a non-invasive marker of the autonomic tone [134].

The above data demonstrate that the mechanism of action of ECP may not be a singular one, but rather a combination of peripheral and cardiac effects. Whether ECP improves the myocardial perfusion and any such improvement is related to collateral growth are subject to controversy [85]. To elucidate the latter hypothesis, the gold standard invasive method to detect the collateral arteries was for the first time investigated in the current trial.

2 The Study's Hypothesis

The objectives of this study were to:

- provide clinical data that arteriogenesis is the main mechanism underlying the beneficial effects of ECP in patients with stable coronary artery disease
- provide clinical data that myocardial blood flow improves after ECP
- assess the link between improvement of the myocardial blood flow and clinical improvement in response to therapy
- investigate possible effects of ECP on coronary microcirculation
- assess the effect of ECP on the left ventricular function

3 Patients and methods

3.1 Study population

This study is the second clinical trial of the Arteriogenesis Network (Art.Net.2). It was designed as a prospective controlled, proof-of-concept study and took place from December 2006 to January 2008. The participating center was the Franz-Volhard-Klinik, Helios Klinikum Berlin-Buch, Charité-Univeristätsmedizin Berlin. The study was conducted in accordance with the principles of the declaration of Helsinki and was approved by the ethical committee of the Charité-Univeristätsmedizin Berlin. Written informed consent was obtained from all patients. A total of 23 patients were recruited between February 2007 and September 2008 in the Department of Cardiology, Franz-Volhard-Klinik, Helios Klinikum Berlin-Buch. All patients were being attended in the out- or in-patient clinic of the hospital.

3.1.1 Inclusion and exclusion criteria

Patients between 40 and 80 years old, who had diagnosed with stable coronary artery disease, were considered for screening. Only patients who were known to have a residual severe, but low risk stenosis of type A according to the AHA/ACC glossary [135, 136] with a positive ischemic stress-test and who were being advised to undergo percutaneous revascularization were considered as probable candidates for the study. An ischemic test was considered as positive if inducible ischemia appeared in myocardial scintigraphy, stress-echocardiography or in cardiac magnetic resonance with stress test (dobutamine or adenosine infusion). Patients whose coronary status were unknown, but who had a positive stress-test and were advised to undergo a diagnostic coronary angiography were also considered for inclusion. To rule out a transmural infarction in the region of interest, cardiac magnetic resonance imaging (CMR) with delayed enhancement was performed on the candidate patients prior to cardiac catheterization. Given that the study participants still met the inclusion criteria, the final decisions to include them or not were made during the cardiac catheterization depending upon the fractional flow reserve (FFR). Only patients who had stable CAD and FFRs less than 0.80 were recruited for the study. In addition to the published contraindications for ECP treatment [99], the exclusion criteria for our study included unstable angina, previous transmural infarction in the area supplied by the narrowed coronary artery (region of interest), as well as contraindications for CMR and administration of adenosine. Furthermore, due to the fact that the therapy took place daily in the outpatient clinic over a period of seven weeks, only patients who were living within a distance of 25 km from the hospital were considered for recruitment. Table 3-1 summarizes the inclusion and exclusion criteria.

Table 3-1: Inclusion and exclusion criteria

Inclusion Criteria

- 40 to 80 years of age
- Stable coronary vessel disease
- Angiographically visual significant stenosis (>70%) of at least one epicardial coronary artery
- Positive imaging stress test (myocardial scintigraphy, stress-echo, adenosine or dobutamine stress cardiac magnetic imaging) for the region of interest (ROI)
- Fractional Flow Reserve (FFR) < 0.80

Exclusion Criteria

- Unstable angina
- Severe kinking of coronary vessels or vessel anatomy unfavorable for pressure measurements
- Magnetic resonance-incompatible metallic implants or known claustrophobia
- Transmural infarction (assessed via CMR) in the area supplied by the narrowed artery
- Ischemic or non-ischemic left ventricle dysfunction with an Ejection Fraction (EF) less than 35%
- Tricuspid and aortic valve insufficiency > moderate and aortic valve stenosis > moderate
- Relevant stenosis of the aorta abdominalis or aorta thoracica, coarctatio aortae
- Atrial fibrillation, severe hypertension with systolic pressure > 180 mmHg
- Symptomatic angiopathy of the lower limb (neuropathy, vasculitis, ankle pressures < 100 mmHg), chronic venous insufficiency > grade III, symptomatic varicosis, thrombosis, occlusion of vena cava inferior, phlebitis
- Lesions of the lower extremity (ulcers, big scar, etc.) or symptomatic orthopedic disease (hip, knee)
- Pre-proliferative or proliferative diabetic retinopathy
- Anticoagulation with International Normalized Ratio (INR) > 3 or INR < 3 and disturbed homeostasis
- Asthma bronchiale, severe systemic disease, pregnancy, mental retardation or dementia
- Acute renal insufficiency, progressive renal insufficiency, chronic renal insufficiency - KDOQI $\geq$ III

3.2 The study design

At the time of the ethics committee approval in 09/2006, the committee gave no permission for inclusion of a sham-ECP or control-group. Hence, the study began with the recruitment of the ECP-group. However, with the publication of the COURAGE Trial [22] that provided evidence that, under optimal medical treatment, PCI can be deferred safely in stable angina pectoris, we received agreement from the ethics committee to include a control-group. Thereafter, all study-participants included were pseudo-randomized in a 2:1 proportion to ECP and control. Since three patients were already in the ECP group, the 4th patient was allocated to the control group and every third patient thereafter was also allocated to the control.

Sixteen patients were prospectively recruited and treated with ECP. Seven patients served as control patients for the natural growth of collateral arteries within seven weeks. The study was conducted in two phases: the pre-study period (phase 1) and the study period (phase 2). Figure 3-1 shows a flow chart of the study.

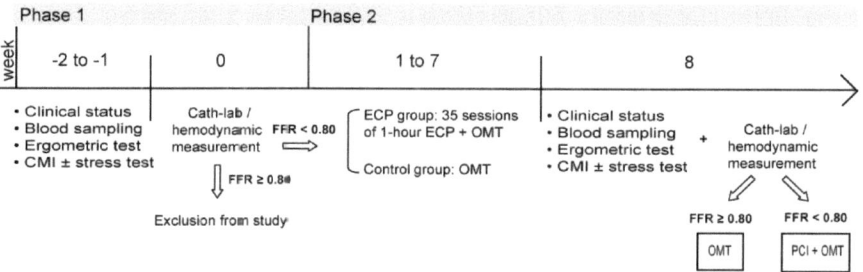

Figure 3-1: *Flow chart of the study (CMI: cardiac magnetic imaging test, OMT: optimal medical therapy, FFR: fractional flow reserve)*

3.2.1.1 Phase One (weeks -2 to 0)

Patients who had stable coronary artery disease and were treated in the in- or out-patient clinic of the participating centre were screened for study eligibility. Potential patients were informed of the study protocol and underwent an ECP test treatment of 30 minutes to confirm that they could tolerate the therapy. After providing written consent, all participants entered the first phase of the trial. Phase one was common to both groups. The clinical symptoms of the patients were assessed twice within two weeks (weeks -2 to -1). The clinical evaluation of the patients was based on standardized questionnaires of the Canadian Cardiovascular Society grading scale (CCS) for angina pectoris and the New York Heart Association (NYHA) functional class for dyspnea at exertion. A questionnaire of the daily physical activities of the patients was completed. Patients were instructed not to modify their daily activities from that point in time until the study protocol had been completed. Oral antihypertensive medication, if not appropriate, was adjusted to meet the guideline recommendations [137]. An echocardiography at baseline was performed. Patients who had not already undergone a myocardial stress-test (scintigraphy imaging, stress-echocardiography or stress perfusion magnetic resonance imaging of the heart) underwent an adenosine stress CMR. If the existence of at least one angiographically significant stenosis of type A according to AHA/ACC [136] was confirmed during the baseline coronary angiography, the hemodynamic significance of the stenosis was evaluated by fractional flow reserve (FFR). Taking into account the fact that all patients had a positive ischemic stress test at the time of catheterization, patients were recruited in the study if FFR<0.80 [21, 138]. If FFR≥0.80 the patient was excluded from the study.

3.2.1.2 Phase Two (weeks 1-8):

In the second phase of the study, patients were divided into the ECP group and the control group. In the ECP group the ECP therapy was undertaken using the standard treatment course, which comprises sixty minutes of therapy five times weekly for a period of seven weeks. At the end of the therapy, each patient had received 35 hours of ECP. Clinical symptoms, blood pressure and heart rate were registered at each treatment session. During the seven-week period, the control group received optimal medical treatment and coaching according to the therapeutic goals within the COURAGE Trial [22]. These included an improvement of clinical symptoms and a reduction of cardiovascular risk factors and poor health behavior. This was accomplished by medical therapy, regular physician surveillance and lifestyle, as well as nutrition counseling by a skilled staff. To compensate for the non-therapy-related effect (increased daily activity in the ECP treatment group due to walk-in treatment, regular contact to the study-team), the control group had an appointment within our clinic five days per week throughout a seven-week period for counseling or non-study-related diagnostics: ultrasound, ankle-brachial index, 24h blood-pressure measurements, ergometric test, 24-hour ECG reading, and a weekly advisory by a dietary consultant. In addition, the control group was seen by the study-physician twice weekly to assess CAD-related symptoms and patients' concerns.

Most antihypertensive medication is known to influence myocardial circulation and deregulate collateral blood flow [139-142]. Therefore, only hydrochlorothiazide was adjusted, if necessary, in both groups [143]. In both groups, concomitant medication was defined as background medication and was kept unchanged in Phase 2. Dose-adjusted lipid-lowering medication was given in both groups. Thus, the known beneficial effect of lipid-lowering medication on the collateral blood flow was expected in both groups [144, 145]. In the 8th week, after having completed the study-course, follow-up with the identical-to-baseline, non-invasive tests and invasive measurements were performed. After assessing the study-related hemodynamic measurements, PCI and stenting was performed or not performed, according to the guidelines [21, 146].

3.3 Clinical endpoints and non-invasive measurements

3.3.1 History and clinical examination

A detailed medical history of each patient was taken in Phase one, before inclusion in the protocol of the study. Data including the following variables were recorded: previous cardiovascular events (infarction, acute coronary syndromes, hospital admissions due to unstable angina, etc), previous cardiovascular interventions and the presence of risk factors for coronary artery disease (hypertension, diabetes, hyperlipidemia, positive family history, and smoking). The CCS grading scale was used to assess angina. The NYHA classification was obtained to assess exercise-induced dyspnea (Table 3-2). The height and weight of each patient was recorded. A general clinical examination and an ECG followed. If necessary, additional tests, such as peripheral artery duplex, were conducted. The medical history, classification of angina/dyspnea and clinical examination were repeated weekly.

Table 3-2: *Evaluation of clinical symptoms*

CCS Classification	NYHA Classification
Class 0: No angina at any level or strength of physical activity	**Class I:** No limitation of physical activity. Ordinary physical activity does not cause undue fatigue, palpitation, or dyspnea (shortness of breath)
Class I: Angina with rapid or strenuous or prolonged exertion only	
Class II: Angina on walking or climbing stairs rapidly, walking uphill or exertion after meals, in cold weather, when under emotional stress, or only during the first hours after awakening	**Class II:** Slight limitation of physical activity. Ordinary physical activity results in fatigue, palpitation, or dyspnea
Class III: Angina on walking one or two blocks on the level or one flight of stairs at a normal pace under normal conditions	**Class III:** Marked limitation of physical activity. Less than ordinary activity causes fatigue, palpitation, or dyspnea
Class IV: Inability to carry out any physical activity without discomfort or "angina at rest"	**Class IV:** Unable to carry out any physical activity without symptoms

3.3.2 Clinical laboratory evaluation

Blood samples were drawn at week 0 and 8. Determination of blood cell counts (hemoglobin, hematocrit, platelet count and white blood cell count), cardiac markers (Troponine-T, CK, CK-MB), haemostatic tests (PTT, prothrombin time, INR), electrolytes, creatinine and lipid profile (total cholesterol, triglycerides, LDL, HDL) were carried out. All blood analyses took place on the same day at the hospital laboratory of Helios Klinikum, Berlin-Buch.

3.3.3 Exercise test

A symptom-limited bicycle ergometric test was performed at baseline (phase 1) and after the ECP therapy (week 8). An ergometric system from General Electric was used (model: Kiss and eBike L). Continuous monitoring of symptoms, 12-canal electrocardiogram and heart rate monitoring were performed. The blood pressure was measured at 2-min intervals. The test started at 50 watts and continued with an increase of 25 watts every two minutes. The examination was terminated due to the emergence of modest to severe angina or dyspnea, exhaustion or presence of other indications, according to the guidelines [147]. The achievable workload, rate-pressure product, exercise duration, maximal heart rate, time-to-occurrence of symptoms, and time and severity of electrocardiographic changes were recorded for the study analysis.

3.3.4 Cardiac magnetic resonance imaging

CMR, including a protocol of delayed enhancement and left ventricular assessment, was performed for all patients in the ECP group at baseline and at week 8. For patients in the control group, the CMR was only performed at baseline. In addition, for patients who presented without an ischemic test, CMR was extended to a stress-test with application of adenosine. For each patient, the same CMR-protocol to the baseline was repeated at week 8. Images were acquired using a 1.5 T magnetic resonance scanner (Sonata, Siemens Medical Solutions, Erlangen, Germany). Localization was performed using breath-hold, single-phase, steady-state, free precession images in 2, 3 and 4 chamber views. Retrospective-gated, steady-state, free precession cine images were then acquired in short axis views covering the left ventricle (slice thickness/gap: 10/0 mm) and in long axis (2-, 3- and 4-chamber) views. Ten minutes after intravascular injection of 0.2 mmol gadolinium-DTPA (Magnevist, Schering, Germany) / kg, late gadolinium enhancement (LGE) images covering the left ventricle were acquired using a standard two-dimensional segmented inversion recovery gradient echo pulse sequence (TR: 5 ms, TE: 1.3, matrix: 256 × 256, field of view 340–380 mm, slice thickness 10 mm with no gap, spatial resolution: 1.3 × 1.3 × 10 mm) with an inversion time optimized to a normal myocardial signal of zero.

Epicardial and endocardial borders of the left ventricle (LV) were traced manually in the stack of short axis cine images at end-systole and end-diastole using commercially available cardiac postprocessing software (MASS Suite ® 6.2.3, Medis, Leiden, Netherlands). Papillary muscles and trabecula were excluded for LV volume determination. Model-free measures of left ventricular diastolic and systolic volumes, ejection fraction, left ventricular mass, stroke volume and cardiac output were calculated.

3.4 Invasive measurements and endpoints

3.4.1 Fractional Flow Reserve (FFR)

The pressure derived fractional flow reserve is an index that allows the functional evaluation of the severity of a stenosis. FFR shows to what extent a particular stenosis affects the myocardial blood flow or the ischemic potential of a stenosis. The method was proposed and established from Pijls and De Bruyne in the past decade [148, 149]. FFR is estimated under maximal hyperemia because it is the maximum flow to meet the metabolic demands of the heart to prevent ischemia. Consequently, FFR is calculated from the ratio of the maximum myocardial blood flow in the presence of a stenosis (Q) to the normal maximum flow (Q_n) (Equation 3-1):

$$\text{Equation 3-1: } FFR = \frac{Q}{Q_n}$$

The Q_n represents the theoretical myocardial flow if no stenosis is present. Q and Q_n are estimated as follows:

$$\text{Equation 3-2: } Q = \frac{(P_d - P_v)}{R} \qquad \text{Equation 3-3: } Q_n = \frac{(P_a - P_v)}{R}$$

where P_d represents the mean hyperemic distal coronary pressure, P_a the mean hyperemic aortic pressure, P_v the mean hyperemic central venous pressure and R the myocardial resistance under maximum vasodilatation.

Assuming that resistance at maximal dilatation is minimal, the next equation can been used to assess the FFR [150]:

$$\text{Equation 3-4: } FFR = \frac{P_d - P_v}{P_a - P_v}$$

The next figure gives an example of this approach:

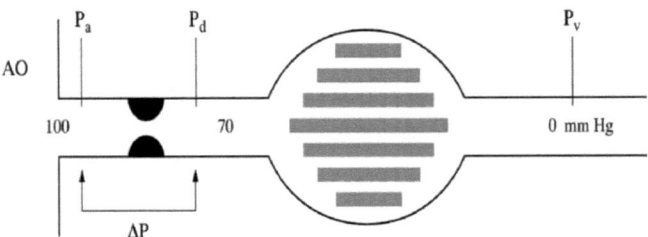

Figure 3-2: *Stenotic coronary artery and the myocardium supplied under maximum hyperemia. In this case, FFR=(70-0)/(100-0)=0.7. A ratio of 0.7 signifies that only 70% of the maximum myocardial blood flow is preserved in the presence of the stenosis. From [151], reproduced with permission from the BMJ Publishing Group.*

In the absence of a stenosis, no pressure gradient exists across the coronary artery and pressure derived-FFR=1. This is the physiological value of a non-diseased coronary artery and undisturbed myocardial distribution. The FFR index is independent of hemodynamic conditions, like heart rate, blood pressure and myocardial contractility, as long as P_d and P_a are measured simultaneously under maximal hyperemia [150]. It is therefore admissible to use the index for inter- and intra-individual comparisons. Furthermore, FFR takes into account the collateral contribution to the myocardial blood flow and any change of the collateral blood flow is reflected in the FFR [61].

The FFR is validated as an accurate method to differentiate whether an epicardial stenosis induces ischemia and must be treated with PCI [138, 149, 152]. An FFR <0.75 indicates a stenosis in need of revascularization. A value greater than 0.80 excludes ischemia in 90% of the cases and is defined as the cut-off point to defer intervention [138, 153, 154]. The last guidelines suggest that a "grey zone" exists for FFR values between 0.75-0.80 in regards to performing or not performing an intervention [21]. However, new data suggest that, when FFR>0.75, the risk of death or myocardial infarction if a PCI is deferred is <1% per year and does not differ from the risk of patients who undergo PCI for an FFR>0.75 [155].

FFR acts in this study-setting as a criterion for inclusion, as well as a secondary endpoint. As long as only patients with hemodynamic significant stenosis are eligible to enter the study, we decided to recruit patients if they fulfilled both following criteria: positive stress-test (as mentioned in chapter 3.1.1) and FFR<0.80. Thus, the decision whether to include a patient was dependent on the FFR-index in the catheterization laboratory.

3.4.2 Collateral flow index (CFIp)

The main hypothesis of the study, that external counterpulsation leads to an improvement of the coronary collateral arteries, was investigated by measurement of the CFIp. The CFIp was the primary endpoint. As previously mentioned, the pressure-derived collateral flow index is currently the gold standard for assessment of collateral blood flow [54].

The CFIp represents the maximum recruitable collateral flow reserve (Qc) as a fraction of the normal myocardial perfusion (Qn):

$$\text{Equation 3-5: } CFIp = \frac{Q_c}{Q_n}$$

In other words, CFIp expresses the blood flow distal to a coronary occlusion that is maintained due to the presence of collateral arteries as a percentage of the normal flow, if the artery was open. The estimate of the index in clinical practice is based on pressure measurements and is calculated in the next equation [150]:

$$\text{Equation 3-6: } CFIp = \frac{P_w - P_v}{P_a - P_v}$$

where P_w represents mean distal coronary pressure during balloon occlusion (coronary wedge pressure), P_a the mean aortic pressure, and P_v the mean central venous pressure.

In other words, the CFIp expresses the percentage of blood pressure distally to an occlusion as part of the blood pressure, if the epicardial coronary artery was not occluded. The distal pressure is dependent on the existence and amount of collateral arteries supplying the post-occluded myocardium with blood. Equation 3-6 can be applied in a model of coronary circulation like that in the next figure:

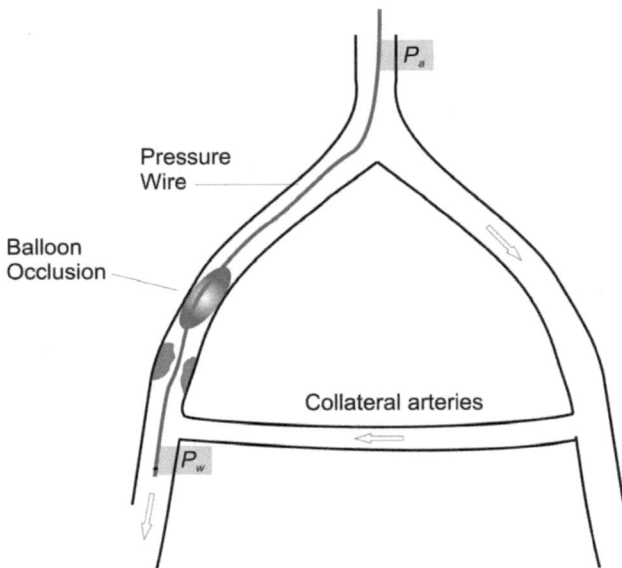

Figure 3-3: *During a brief balloon occlusion proximally to the stenosis, the distal "wedge" pressure (Pw) is measured by the pressure wire. Pa is measured by the guide wire in the aorta. Pw depends on blood supply by the collateral arteries.*

To estimate the contribution of the collateral arteries to coronary perfusion, it is essential that the antegrade flow is interrupted. This interruption can be performed artificially by a brief coronary occlusion, as in Figure 3-3. In our study the pressure measurements were not performed in occluded vessels, but in coronary arteries that had at least one significant stenosis. In this case, to measure the wedge pressure, a brief occlusion of 60-70s was performed by carefully inflating a PCI-balloon proximally to the stenosis of interest in order to interrupt the antegrade flow. During the occlusion P_a, P_w and P_v were simultaneously recorded. The short-term coronary occlusion serves not only the block of the antegrade coronary flow, but also is the ischemic stimulus for recruitment of collateral arteries. It has been suggested that the 60-70 second duration of the balloon inflation is sufficient for maximal recruitment of collaterals without causing any harm to the myocardium [60].

3.4.3 Index of microcirculatory resistance (IMR)

Another important issue that remained unclear was whether ECP exerts any effects on the microcirculation of the heart. A method to assess the microcirculation is to evaluate the ability of these small vessels to vasodilate and induce a subsequent increase of coronary blood flow. The small vessels (<400μm) are the main source of resistance to flow [156] and upon vasodilatation, for example with adenosine, they contribute maximally to increased coronary blood flow. The magnitude of the increase in coronary blood flow under hyperemia (from basal coronary perfusion to maximal coronary vasodilatation) is termed coronary flow reserve (CFR) [157]. Pijls and De Bruyne introduced a method to measure CFR simultaneously with the pressure measurements necessary for the calculation of FFR by using the principles of thermodilution [158, 159]. The commercially available guidewire for intracoronary pressure measurements (PressureWire, Radi Medical Systems) is equipped with a sensor on its tip, measuring pressure and temperature simultaneously. The shaft of the wire can recognize the start of a saline injection and act, therefore, as a proximal "thermo sensor." By injecting a bolus of saline through the guiding catheter at a temperature lower than that of blood, it is possible to measure the "traveling time" of the injectate (saline) from the guiding catheter to the distal sensor. This is referred as transit mean time (Tmn). Thus, Tmn shows how fast the injectate flows in the coronary arteries. It is dependent on the coronary resistance. By measuring the Tmn at rest and under hyperemia, it is possible to assess the increase in the coronary blood flow as a result of the reduction of resistance, mainly of the distal small arteries. In this case, the CFR is calculated from the following equations:

Equation 3-7: $CFR = \dfrac{Fhyperemia}{Frest} \Rightarrow CFR = \dfrac{\left(\dfrac{V}{Tmn}\right)hyperemia}{\left(\dfrac{V}{Tmn}\right)rest} \Rightarrow CFR = \dfrac{(Tmn)rest}{(Tmn)hyperemia}$

F and V represent blood flow and coronary volume respectively. For further information about the mathematical approach, we refer to the related articles [158, 159].

Although CFR is a useful index to assess coronary microvascular resistance in the absence of CAD, it has only a limited accuracy when an epicardial stenosis occurs. Furthermore, CFR depends on the hemodynamic, like heart rate, making serial measurements difficult to compare [160, 161].

Since, in our study, patients who had significant epicardial stenosis were recruited, another index of microcirculation, the microcirculatory resistance index (IMR), which is independent of the severity of an epicardial stenosis [162, 163] was chosen. IMR is calculated from P_d and Tmn obtained under hyperemia as follows:

$$\text{Equation 3-8: } IMR = P_d \times T_{mn}$$

IMR is believed to be independent of hemodynamics. Both Pd and Tmn are simultaneously measured under maximal hyperemia, thereby eliminating the dependence on rest conditions as is the case with CFR. Although IMR generally does not depend on an epicardial stenosis, the presence of collateral arteries would increase P_d and lead to an overestimation of the index. In this case, Equation 3-8 must be modified to take the collateral blood supply into account. A pre-requisite for this is that a coronary occlusion or wedge pressure (P_w) be known [164]:

$$\text{Equation 3-9: } IMRcor = P_a \times T_{mn} \times (\frac{P_d - P_w}{P_a - P_w})$$

P_a, P_d and Tmn are estimated under maximal vasodilatation, whereas P_w is obtained under a brief coronary occlusion. The last equation was used for the off-line calculation of the IMR in the present study. All parameters of the equation were obtained during the coronary catheterization as described in the next chapters. To avoid confusion with the terminology when referring to numerical values, the simple term IMR will be used from now on for values based on the simple equation 3-8 and the term IMRcor. for results from equation 3-9.

To evaluate the effect of hemodynamic loading conditions, the central venous pressure is taken into account when calculating the IMR. To date it has only been hypothesized that central venous pressure can be excluded from the IMR calculation. In the current trial we measured all parameters needed directly for an accurate estimate of the microcirculation resistance. So, we assessed IMR by taking the venous pressure into account in the next equation [162] :

$$\text{Equation 3-10: } IMRcvp = (Pa - Pv) \cdot Tmn \cdot \left(\frac{Pd - Pw}{Pa - Pw}\right)$$

Based on earlier studies of thermodilution [159, 165], we calculated the variability between each set of three transit mean times as:

Equation 3-11: $Var(a1, a2, a3) = \max(i = 1,2,3) \cdot \dfrac{|ai - \overline{a}|}{\overline{a}}$

3.4.4 Quantitative coronary angiography

At week 0 and 8, standard diagnostic angiography was performed before the invasive measurements. QCA was performed in order to exclude possible changes in the stenosis severity during the study period that could influence the functional data acquired. The angiographic data were digitalized, collected and analyzed. All angiograms had to meet appropriate standards for quantitative angiographic imaging. Before the measurements, the target vessel was imaged in identical projections (orthogonal where possible) and at magnifications (> 2 for the right coronary artery [RCA] or > 3 for the left circumflex artery [LCX] and the left anterior descending artery [LAD]) that appeared suitable for a QCA analysis (CAAS II, Pie Medical System, Maastricht, Netherlands). Coronary artery stenoses were assessed quantitatively as the percent of reduction in diameter using the guiding catheter for calibration.

3.4.5 Protocol of cardiac catheterization and invasive measurements

Invasive procedures were performed in the catheterization laboratory of the Franz-Volhard-Klinik, Charité-Universitätsmedizin in Berlin. The procedure was performed on a standard angiography suite (Hicor, Siemens, Erlangen, Germany). The pressures were measured in mm Hg. The aortic pressure (P_a) was measured in the ascending aorta by the guiding catheter. The venous pressure (P_v) was measured with a catheter placed in the right atrium. Pressures distal to the stenosis (P_d or P_w) and thermodilution curves were obtained by using the PressureWire® 5 or PressureWire® Certus (Radi Medical systems, Uppsala, Sweden). The PressureWire® is a 0.014" guidewire with a length of 175 cm. A high fidelity sensor is located 3 cm proximal to its radiopaque tip. The sensor is suitable for simultaneously pressure and temperature measurements within an operating range of -30 to +300 mm Hg and 15-42^{0}C. The wire is connected to a device (RadiAnalyzer® Express), which enables a real time display of measurements, an automatic calculation of FFR and the storage of the data. The device is connected to the catheterization system for calibration and equalization of the catheters and a bidirectional transfer of pressure-data.

Steady state hyperemia for assessment of FFR and IMR was achieved by administration of adenosine (Adenoscan® 30mg/10ml, Sanofi-Aventis) through a large antecubital vein at a rate of 140μg kg^{-1} min^{-1} [166]. The hyperemic measurements were begun after adenosine had been administered for two minutes and continued during the infusion for one to two minutes in order to complete the study's protocol.

3.4.6 Performance of the invasive measurements

During catheterization, the patient was under continuous ECG and blood pressure monitoring. The right femoral approach was used in all patients. After sterilization and application of local anesthesia with lidocaine, the femoral artery was punctured and a right or left 6-French (F) guiding catheter without side holes was inserted and advanced initially to the left ventricle for measurement of the left ventricular end-diastolic pressure. Next, a 5F catheter was inserted into the femoral vein and advanced into the right atrium to record the Pv. Weight adjusted heparin was administered intravenously. 0.2 mg of nitroglycerine was given intracoronary and repeated, if needed, every 25 minutes throughout the cardiac catheterization to prevent any occurrence of coronary spasm due to the injection of contrast agent. Diagnostic angiography of the target vessel, or of all three coronary arteries, was performed as indicated above (see Chapter 3.4.4). If by angiography, the known stenosis was characterized as significant, but low-risk type A stenosis [136], the procedure was continued with the pressure measurements. An interval of 10-minutes was allowed for dissipation of the effect of the non-ionic contrast agent on the coronary vasomotion.

The pressure wire was set to zero, calibrated and advanced to the tip of the guiding catheter to ensure that the pressures recorded by the guiding catheter and the pressure wire were identical. If a pressure difference was detected, this was removed by equalizing the pressures. Thereafter, the wire was advanced through the guiding catheter distal to the stenosis [59]. The measurements were started with three injections of 3 ml of saline into the guiding catheter. A deviation of < 15% of Tmean was accepted for analysis of the Tmean. Subsequently, the administration of adenosine was initiated and two minutes for steady state hyperemia were allowed. Under continuous administration of adenosine, the three saline injections were repeated. Thermodilution curves, transit mean times (Tmn) and pressure values at rest and under hyperemia were recorded. After the measurements, the FFR value was displayed. If FFR>0.80 the patient was not eligible for inclusion and the study protocol was terminated. Further diagnostic or therapeutic procedures for these patients were performed, if needed, independently of the study protocol.

If FFR<0.80, the patient was recruited into the study and the study protocol was continued with the assessment of the CFIp. An adequately sized PCI-balloon was advanced over the pressure wire and placed right proximal to the stenosis. The pressure wire was not removed and remained steady distal to the stenosis. The balloon was inflated at a low pressure (1-3 atm) until the antegrade coronary flow was interrupted. This was checked with an injection of contrast dye. The balloon remained inflated for 60-70s and all three pressures (P_a, P_w, P_v) were displayed and recorded continuously. The balloon could be deflated earlier if a patient developed excessive angina symptoms or ST-elevations were recorded in the ECG. After deflation of the balloon, sufficient time was allowed for normalization of the pressures to the output values. The vessel was examined for a possible dissection. If no complication occurred, the patient was discharged from the hospital on the following day.

The same protocol was repeated after completion of the ECP therapy in week 8. During this catheterization and after the FFR and CFIp measurements, the decision to treat the stenosis with PCI/stent was made. Taking into account the clinical status of the patient, the non-invasive stress test, the FFR measurement and the guidelines [21], an intervention was performed for all FFR values under 0.75 and most of the patients with 0.75<FFR<0.80. If in week 8, the FFR was greater than 0.80, no intervention was performed.

3.4.7 Calculation of the invasive endpoints

The FFR index was automatically displayed in the monitor during the cardiac catheterization. These values were used to provide information about study inclusion/exclusion and whether to conduct a PCI. All four invasive endpoints were calculated blind offline at the end of the study.

FFR was estimated as the mean value of the three pressure loops that were registered during application of saline during hyperemia. In each of these three loops, the minimal Pa and Pd values estimated after at least three adjacent heart beats free of artifacts (e.g., due to breath), and in the absence of any extra systole, were considered for the final calculation of the FFR.

The three lowest pressures of the last 10 seconds of the balloon occlusion, namely the seconds 60-70 values (Pa, Pw, Pv) were chosen for the calculation of CFIp (curves with artifacts were excluded). If a patient had a shorter balloon occlusion in one or both examinations due to excessive angina or to ST-elevations, the CFIp calculation was based on the last 10 seconds of the shorter duration of occlusion (e.g., between 30-40 s for an occlusion of 40 s). Thereafter, the CFIp on the other time point (week 0 or week 8) was calculated at the same time interval (e.g. 30-40 s) despite the fact that a longer coronary occlusion might be available.

IMR/IMRcor. were calculated from the pressure values that were obtained for the estimation of the FFR (Pa and Pd) and CFIp (Pw). The mean value of the three registered Tmns under hyperemia was taken as transit mean time (Tmn).

3.5 External Counterpulsation therapy (ECP)

The ECP treatments took place on five days per week from week 1 to week 7 for a total of 35 hours of therapy. Every session lasted one hour. Clinical symptoms and adverse experiences (like cramps or aching muscles) during the preceding 24 hours were recorded at each treatment session. Vital signs (blood pressure, heart rate) were also recorded and legs were examined for areas of redness or ecchymosis. The TS3 device (Vasomedical Inc., Westbury, New York) was used for the external counterpulsation therapy. The equipment consists of a console with an air-compressor, a treatment table and three pairs of cuffs. After the cuffs are wrapped around the calves, lower and upper thighs, they are compressed with air in a sequence synchronized with the cardiac cycle. The heart rhythm of the patient is conducted through a 3-canal ECG. Blood pressure waveforms are monitored during ECP by finger plethysmography. From these waveforms, the D/S ratio, an index of the hemodynamic effect of ECP, is estimated. The D/S ratio or ECP effectiveness ratio was calculated as the ratio of the peak diastolic amplitude divided by the peak systolic amplitude averaged over five cardiac cycles. External counterpulsation was performed at cuff pressures ranging from 200 to 260 mm Hg depending on the patient's tolerance of the therapy and the achieved hemodynamic effect with a target D/S ratio of 1.0-1.5 [96].

3.6 Sample size and Statistical analysis

The strongest evidence for ECP-related improvement of myocardial blood flow due to adaptive collateral arterial growth is provided by former PET studies [109, 167]. PET (sensitivity >90% and specificity >80% respectively for CAD) [168] is considered to be a reliable method to non-invasively detect coronary collaterals (sensitivity up to 90%, specificity up to 88% and accuracy up to 90%) [169]. The methodological error of CFIp and FFR measurement was taken into account by reviewing prospective trials [67, 138, 150].

The power calculations are based on the aforementioned studies reporting perfusion changes after ECP treatment and the following assumptions: One-tailed test for increase in myocardial blood flow in the ischemic region, significance level of 5 %, desired power to detect change 80%, a mean change of myocardial blood flow respectively collateral blood flow in ischemic myocardial region of at least + 15 %. These assumptions are similar to other estimates of significant increases of perfusion after ECP treatment detected primarily by SPECT.

Based on these assumptions, a sample size of 12 patients was required for the ECP group. Assuming a drop-out rate of 30-40%, it was planned to include a total of 18 patients. In the ECP group, recruitment was finished as soon as 16 patients were included. Because a reduced variance had been observed in published data on the natural course of the collateral circulation, a 2:1 ratio for the control group was planned, resulting in a sample size of 7 patients (6 + 1 expected drop out).

Intra-individual comparisons of baseline data versus follow-up data were conducted using the paired Student t-test and Wilcoxon test. Between-group comparisons of continuous clinical, hemodynamic, angiographic, and fractional flow and collateral flow data were performed by t-test and ANOVA or Mann-Whitney-test and Friedman-test.

A chi^2 test using Fishers exact test was applied for a comparison of categorical variables among the two study groups. A linear regression analysis was performed to assess the association between the D/S ratio and the invasive endpoints. Data are presented as means ± standard deviation in the text or as means ± standard error in the figures. Statistical significance was defined as $p < 0.05$. All analyses were calculated using the software package SPSS 15.0.

4 Results

4.1 Patients

From December 2006 to May 2008, about 622 records of patients with CAD from the database of the Franz-Volhard-Klinik were examined for eligibility for recruitment into the study. Forty of the 600 patients were considered as eligible for inclusion and were contacted and informed about the clinical trial. After the baseline diagnostic tests (ischemic stress test and CMR or stress CMR) and the FFR measurements, 23 patients were finally included. Sixteen patients were allocated to the ECP group and seven patients to the control group. No patient withdrew after enrollment in the trial.

4.1.1 Characteristics of the study population

A total of seventeen men and six women were recruited. The mean age of the patients was 61 years (41 to 77 years). The cardiac risk factor profile was high as each patient had at least two risk factors for cardiovascular disease. In total, all patients had hypertension, 22/23 had dyslipidemia and every fourth patient had a positive family history of coronary heart disease. Two patients in every group had diabetes. No differences in any baseline characteristics were seen between the groups (Table 4-1).

The baseline CAD-related medical histories of the patients are presented in Table 4-2. The characterization of the entire coronary status was made visually and only stenoses >50% were taken into account. Most of the patients had a multivessel disease when they were included in the study. The vessel measured through FFR (ROI) was the LAD in 63% of the ECP group and 85% of the control group. About half of the patients in each group had suffered a myocardial infarction in the past and over 80% of the patients had undergone a coronary intervention. There were no statistical differences between the groups in regards to these characteristics.

The daily activity of the patients prior to study inclusion was assessed and patients were classified into two groups. If they had any regular activity (walking or jogging or bicycling or any art of training for more than 30 minutes per day) for more than 5 times per week, they were classified in the "physically active" group (n=12). All other patients were grouped in the sedentary group (n=11). There was no difference between the ECP group and the control group in relation to this characteristic.

Table 4-1: Baseline data of the patients

Category	Subcategory	ECP (n=16)	Control (n=7)	p-value
Demographic characteristics	Age, years (range)	62.3 (43-77)	61.4 (41-75)	0.87
	Male gender, n (%)	11(68.8)	6(85.7)	0.62
	BMI (kg/m^2)	28.5±1.03	28.1±1.25	0.84
Cardiovascular risk factors	Hypertension, n (%)	16(100)	7(100)	-
	Hyperlipidemia, n (%)	15(93.8)	7(100)	1.0
	Diabetes, n (%)	2(12.5)	2(28.5)	0.55
	Family history for CAD, n (%)	4 (25)	2 (28.6)	1.0
	Ongoing smoking, n (%)	3 (18.8)	1 (14.3)	1.0
Cardiac history and current status	Prior myocardial infarct, n (%)	8 (50)	3 (42.9)	1.0
	Prior percutaneous intervention, n (%)	13 (81.3)	6 (85.7)	1.0
	Prior CABG, n (%)	1 (6.3)	0 (0)	1.0
	Ejection fraction (echocardiography), %	62±1.72	58±1.25	0.11
	Systolic blood pressure, mmHg	122±2.81	120±7.15	0.77
	Diastolic blood pressure, mmHg	70±1.76	72±3.4	0.69
	Angina pectoris CCS class 0/ I/ II/ III (%)	56/13/25/6	43/14/29/14	0.91
	NYHA Class I/ II/ III (%)	25/63/12	43/43/14	0.82
	Physical active, n (%)	8 (50)	4 (57.1)	1.0
Baseline stress test	SPECT/ CMR/ Stress echocardiography	3/11/2	2/4/1	-
Blood results	Total cholesterol, mg/dl	173±15.7	162±12.2	0.65
	LDL, mg/dl	101±11.3	90±12.5	0.53
	HDL, mg/dl	47.4±4	49.4±9.8	0.82
	CRP, mg/dl	2.2±0.86	1.43±0.72	0.69

BMI=body-mass index, CABG=coronary artery bypass graft, CCS=Canadian Cardiovascular Society, CMR= cardiac magnetic resonance, CRP=C-reactive protein, ECP=external counterpulsation, HDL=high-density lipoprotein, LDL=low-density lipoprotein, NYHA=New York Heart Association, SPECT=Single Photon Emission Computed Tomography

Table 4-2: CAD history at baseline			
	ECP (n=16)	Control (n=7)	p-value
1-, 2-, 3-vessel disease	6/8/2 (37/50/13 %)	1/2/4 (14/29/57 %)	0.12
lesion of interest (ROI) – LAD/RCA/LCX	10/4/2 (63/25/12 %)	6/1/0 (85/15/0 %)	0.64
previous myocardial infarction	8 (50%)	3 (43%)	1.0
previous intervention (PCI)	13 (81%)	6 (86%)	1.0
number of previous PCIs – 1/2/3/4	8/2/0/3 (62/15/0/23 %)	3/0/2/1 (50/0/33/17 %)	0.26
previous CABG	1 (6%)	0 (0%)	1.0

LAD: left anterior descending artery, LCx: left circumflex artery, RCA: right coronary artery

4.1.2 Adverse events and compliance

No major adverse events occurred during the study due to the invasive and noninvasive diagnostic and interventional procedures. Minor adverse events were observed. For example, paresthesia of the foot during the counterpulsation therapy was reported by four patients. With a brief (two-minute) deactivation of the lowest cuffs on the calves, there was a rapid relief of the symptom. The therapy could be continued without further symptoms. Three patients complained about sore muscles after the therapy. However, the symptoms "faded" without specific treatment within 2-3 hours and no break in the course of the therapy or prescription of medication was needed.

4.2 Endpoints at baseline

4.2.1 Clinical characteristics of the patients

In Phase one, the participants were seen twice within two weeks to ensure that angina was stable and to prompt a stress-test if no recent testing was available. Each patient performed an ergometric test to determine his or her blood pressure profile, the ischemic threshold, or symptom limited stress level. Blood pressure measurements, lipid profiles and clinical statuses were obtained during this pre-study period. Based on these parameters, the medication was adapted. From this point on, the medication was not changed further. Most patients had an "optimal" well balanced medication for the treatment of CAD according to the guidelines [14]. All patients (100%) were on aspirin, β-blocker and a statin. Table 4-3 lists the medications taken at baseline (week 0), reflecting a high use of multiple evidence-based therapies and good compliance by the patients. There was a remarkably low use of nitrates in each group, although 44% of the ECP group and 57% of the control patients experienced effort angina at baseline. Nitroglycerine on request was the only medication that could be adapted to personal needs during the trial.

Table 4-3: Medication at baseline			
	ECP (n=16)	**Control (n=7)**	**p-value**
Aspirin, n (%)	16 (100)	7 (100)	-
Beta-blocker, n (%)	16 (100)	7 (100)	-
ACE inhibitor, n (%)	12 (75)	6 (85.7)	1.0
AT1- antagonist	5 (31.3)	1 (14.3)	0.62
Calcium- antagonist, n (%)	5 (31.3)	1 (14.3)	0.62
Diuretic, n (%)	10 (62.5)	5 (71.4)	1.0
Statin, n (%)	16 (100)	7 (100)	-
Clopidogrel, n(%)	8 (50)	4 (42.9)	1.0
Nitrates, n (%)	2 (28.6)	3 (18.8)	0.62

ACE:angiotensin converting enzyme, AT:angiotensin

Systolic and diastolic blood pressure values were within the optimal range as recommended for the secondary prevention of CAD in both groups and did not differ between the groups at baseline [14, 170]. These values may possibly mirror the intensive medical treatment and good compliance by the patients to the medication. The level of LDL in serum, although varying within the normal range, was optimal (<70mg/dl) only in five patients of the ECP group and in three patients of the control group. All values are presented in Table 4-1.

Angina symptoms were registered daily in the ECP group. In both groups, the symptoms were classified according to the CCS and NYHA classification weekly. In total, 50% of the patients were free of angina at baseline. No statistical difference between the groups in the CCS and NYHA classifications was observed. Females in the ECP group had more severe angina at baseline than males of the ECP group (p=0.002). More than half of the patients in each group reported dyspnea and fatigue at exertion at baseline. There was no gender- or group-related difference in relation to NYHA.

4.2.2 Hemodynamic effect of ECP

The signal in finger plethysmography that is used for the automatic calculation of the D/S ratio is influenced by different factors. The surrounding temperature, the position of the finger relative to the heart level or a pre-constriction of the finger arteries due to excitement or stress can influence blood flow to the finger and, subsequently, the plethysmographic signal [171]. To limit the influence of the parameters on the results, we calculated the D/S ratio at baseline as the mean value of the maximal D/S ratio of the first and fifth sessions. Post ECP, the D/S ratio was the mean value of the maximal D/S ratio during the last three sessions. At baseline, D/S was 0.86±0.06. There was no statistical difference between men (D/S=0.85±0.09) and women (D/S=0.91±0.10).

4.2.3 Non-invasive diagnostic tests at baseline

4.2.3.1 Exercise test

Twenty-one of the 23 patients underwent a bicycle exercise test as described above (see Chapter 3.3.3). One patient had a left brunch bundle block rendering the analysis of the ST-segments impossible. Patients in both groups achieved, on average, 105 watts before stopping the test. No statistical difference in any of the documented parameters of the test was seen between the groups at baseline. However, the ECP group patients tended to achieve higher maximal heart rates (120±4bpm) than the control patients (104±7bpm, p=0.05). All results are presented in Table 4-4.

Table 4-4: Exercise test at baseline			
	ECP	Control	p-value
duration of exercise (sec)	416±28	381±64	0.19
maximal power (Watt)	107±6	103±16	0.76
rate-pressure product (mmHg•bpm)	23983±1293	20237±2394	0.14
maximal heart rate (bpm)	120±4	104±7	0.05

4.2.3.2 Cardiac magnetic resonance

Patients in the ECP and control group underwent CMR for assessment of the left ventricular function and structure at baseline. In Figure 4-1, short images of a patient at diastole and systole are presented. No difference between the groups was seen at baseline. All patients had a normal left ventricular ejection fraction. All results are presented in Table 4-5.

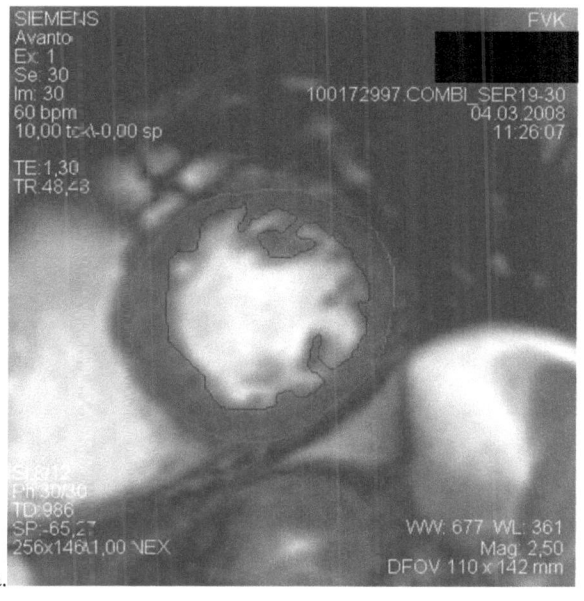

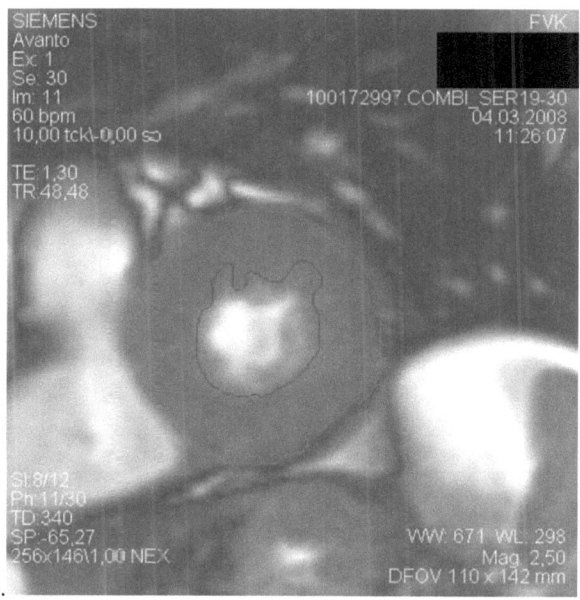

Figure 4-1: *Short axis image of a patient at end-diastole (a) and end-systole (b). The epicardial and endocardial contours are depicted.*

Table 4-5: CMR data on baseline

	ECP	Control	p-value
EF (%)	63±7.2	62±3.4	0.9
ED volume (ml)	151±21	142±24	0.57
LV mass ED (g)	89±24	86±34	0.86
Stroke volume (ml)	94±11	89±11	0.46
Cardiac output (l/min)	6.4±0.8	5.9±0.9	0.45

EF: ejection fraction, ED: end-diastolic, LV: left ventricle

4.2.4 Invasive endpoints at baseline

The evaluation of the primary invasive endpoints at baseline demonstrated that patients in both groups had poor collateral arteries (CFIp<0.25). The ECP group had a lower CFIp=0.08±0.01 than the controls: CFIp=0.15±0.03 (p=0.016). The FFR values did not differ between the groups. The quantitative angiography demonstrated a percent diameter stenosis of 52% and 54% in the ECP group and the control group respectively. The index of microcirculatory resistance (IMR) did not differ between groups. All invasive results at baseline are presented in Table 4-6.

In Figures 4-2 and 4-3 the coronary angiogram and a print-out of the pressure measurements of a patient are presented.

Table 4-6: Baseline angiographic and hemodynamic data

	ECP	Control	p-value
Diameter stenosis of ROI, (%)	52.4±3.46	54.2±4.3	0.76
Fractional flow reserve (FFR), no unit	0.68±0.03	0.68±0.05	0.89
Left ventricular end-diastolic pressure, mmHg	11.6±0.72	13.5±1.5	0.21
Mean aortic pressure at occlusion (Pa), mmHg	89.8±3.86	91.3±3.61	0.82
Coronary occlusive pressure (Pw), mmHg	10.2±1.38	17±2.77	0.025*
CVP during occlusion, mmHg	3.79±0.59	5.25±1.56	0.29
Collateral flow index (CFIp), no unit	0.08±0.01	0.15±0.03	0.016*
Index of microcirculatory resistance (IMRcor) mmHg sec	14.2±2.4	10.1±2.4	0.08

*p<0.05, CVP=central venous pressure, ECP=external counterpulsation, LAD=left anterior descending artery, LCX=left circumflex artery, RCA=right coronary artery, ROI=region of interest

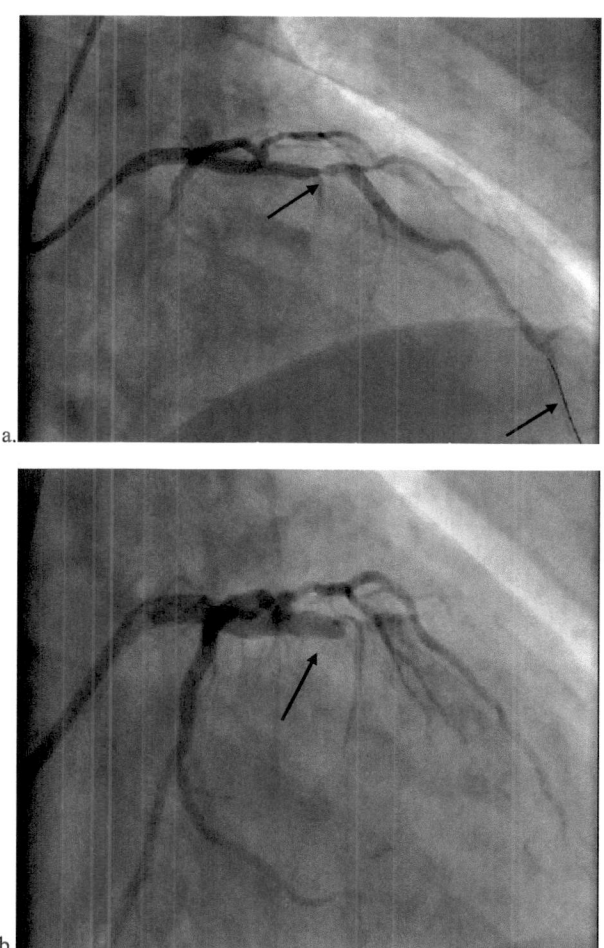

Figure 4-2: *Right anterior oblique (RAO) projection of the LAD of a patient before (a) and during the balloon occlusion (b). The black arrow in picture (a) shows the stenosis and the red arrow the pressure wire which has been placed distally to the stenosis. In picture (b) the balloon is marked by the arrow.*

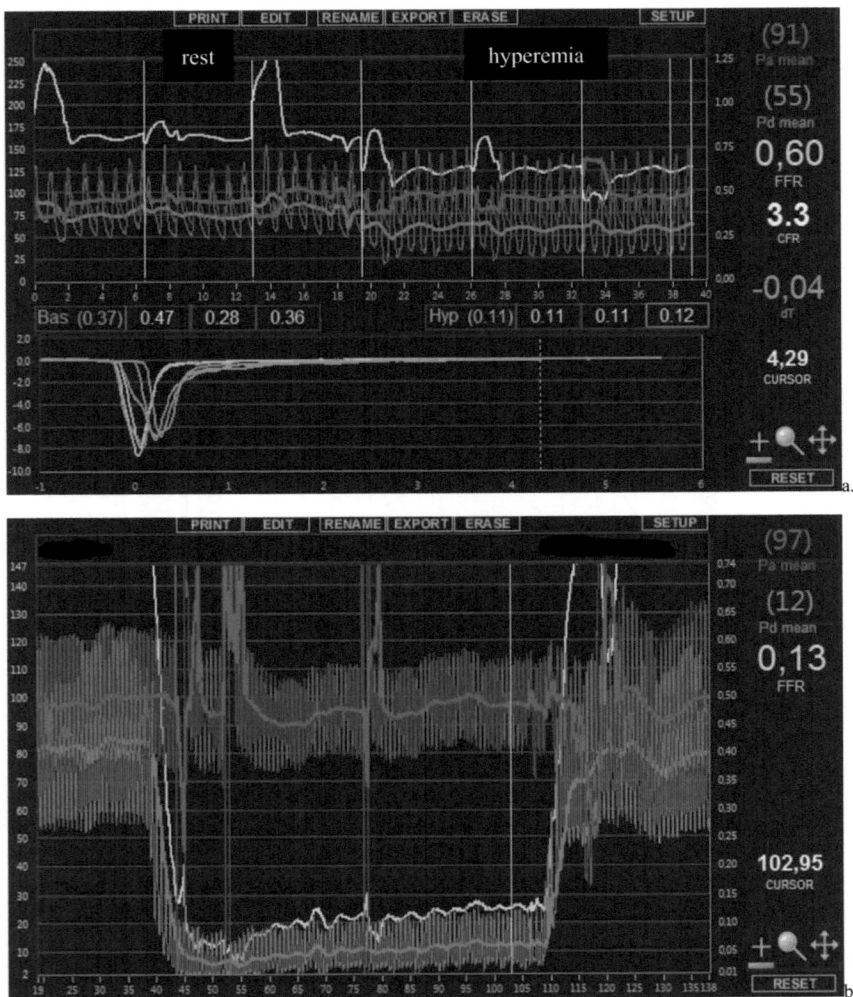

Figure 4-3: *Print-out (from the Radi-View program) of the pressure curves during the three thermodilution measurements at rest and during hyperemia (a). In figure (b) the pressure curves before, during and after the balloon occlusion of the same patient are presented.*

4.3 Endpoints at week 8

4.3.1 Clinical endpoints

A significant reduction of the CCS classification was achieved (p=0.008) in the ECP-group after treatment, whereas no change (p=0.25) was observed in the control group. The severity of dyspnea (NYHA scale) was reduced after ECP (p<0.001) but not within the control (p=0.28). At the conclusion of the therapy, 81% of the ECP patients were free of angina pectoris (CCS=0) compared to 56% at baseline. Among the ECP patients who reported angina at baseline, 66% had a decrease of one CCS class and 34% had a decrease of two classes after ECP. No patient who had been treated with ECP had an increase in angina class or remained in CCS > II after the therapy (figure 4-4). There was no change for the worse in the NYHA classification for any of the patients in the ECP group.

Figures 4-4 and 4-5 present the changes of the CCS and NYHA classifications of both groups during the study period of eight weeks. Although there was a gradual improvement in angina and dyspnea at exertion throughout the ECP therapy, a significant improvement for both the CCS and NYHA scores was seen only at the end of the 7-week therapy course. For CCS, a significant improvement was already seen in the second half of the treatment period.

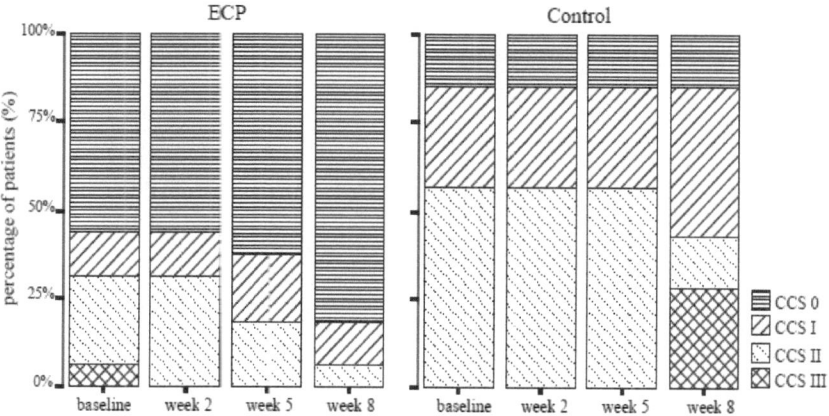

Figure 4-4: *Change of CCS from baseline to week 8*

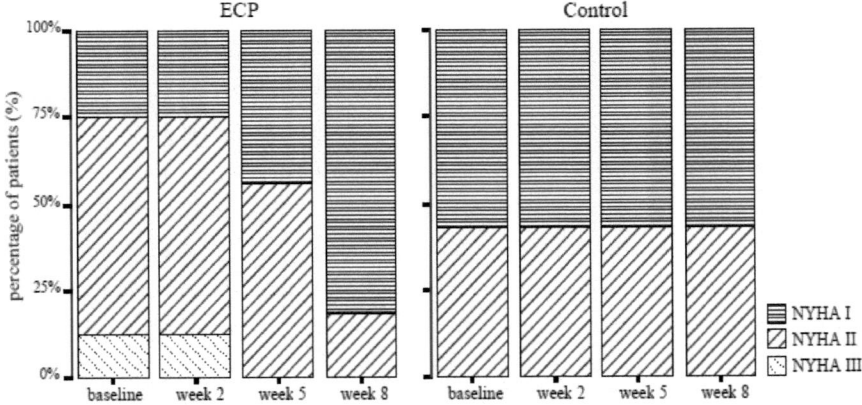

Figure 4-5: *Change of NYHA from baseline to week 8*

The baseline differences between males and females in the CCS classification disappeared in the course of the ECP. After ECP no difference in the CCS scale between males and females was seen. As mentioned above, both males and females had a significant improvement in the CCS and NYHA classification. In a comparison of the relative improvements in the CCS scale between the groups, the females showed a significantly greater change from week 0 to week 8 than did the males (p=0.001). In regard to the change of NYHA scores, there was no difference between males and females.

There was no effect of the therapy on the systolic or diastolic blood pressure values in any of the groups or between the groups and at any point in time. Figure 4-6 presents the blood pressure curves throughout the study period.

The laboratory parameters including the lipid-profile (cholesterol, LDL, HDL) showed no change from baseline to week 8.

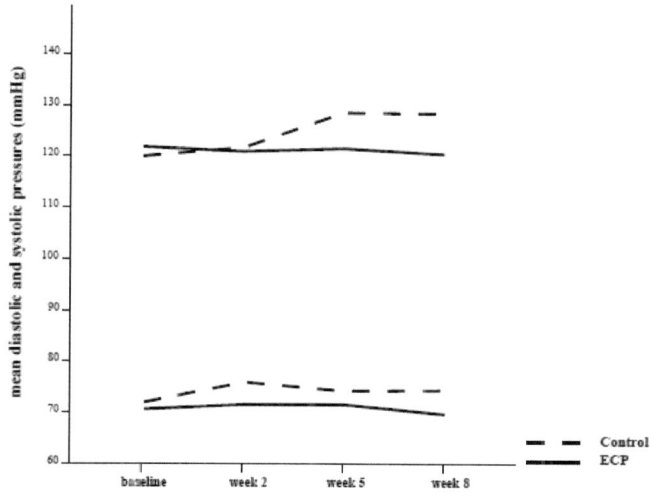

Figure 4-6: *Blood pressure values from week 0 to week 8. There is no statistical difference at any point in time between or inside the groups.*

4.3.2 Specific hemodynamic parameters

The D/S ratio showed a significant improvement throughout the therapy. The mean D/S ratio increased from baseline 0.86±0.06 to 1.07±0.08 at week 9 (p<0.0001, figure 4-7). The improvement in FFR correlated significantly with the improvement in the D/S ratio (p=0.001, r=0.54). There was no statistically significant correlation between the ΔD/S ratio and ΔCFIp (p=0.06). Only patients with an improvement in the CFIp (CFIp-responders) or an improvement in the FFR (FFR-responders) showed a significant increase in the D/S ratio as shown in Figure 4-8.

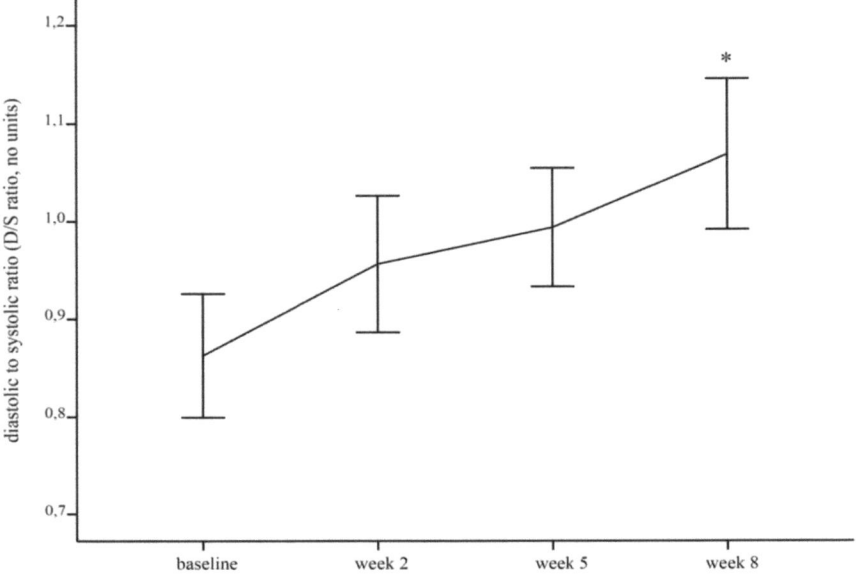

Figure 4-7: *Change in the D/S ratio during the ECP therapy, *p<0.0001*

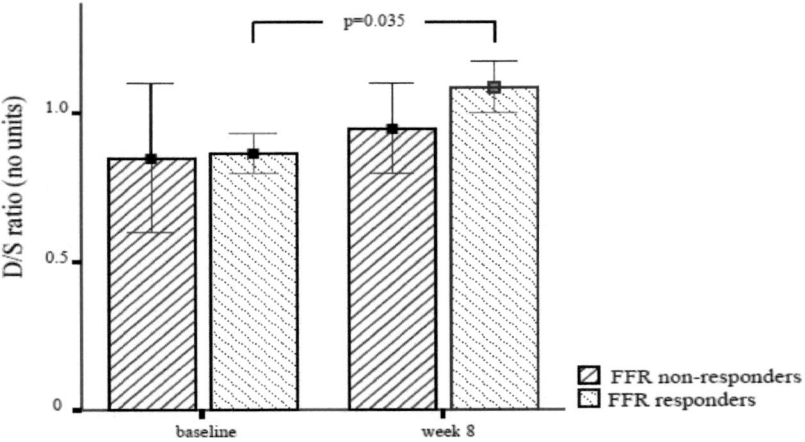

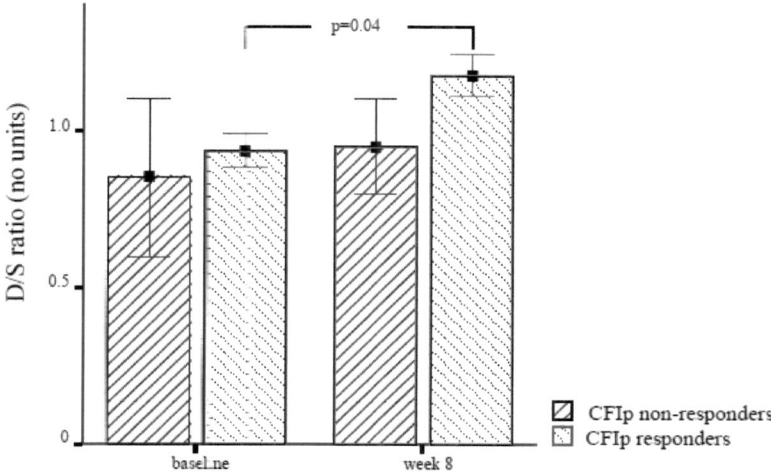

Figure 4-8: *Change in the D/S ratio in relation to the response to CFIp and FFR*

4.3.3 Exercise test

The results of the exercise tests are presented in Table 4-7. There was no statistically significant difference in any of the evaluated parameters. The ECP-group tended to attain at week 8, and also at baseline, a higher heart rate than the control patients (p=0.06).

We must mention that the results of the exercise test may be of limited value as long as 60% of ECP patients and 50% of control patients had stopped the ergometric test due to peripheral exhaustion or orthopedic complaints.

Table 4-7: Results of exercise test						
	ECP			Control		
	baseline	week 8	p-value	baseline	week 8	p-value
duration of exercise (sec)	416±28	423±26	0.78	381±70	360±61	0.3
maximal power (Watt)	107±6	115±7	0.16	103±16	100±13	0.31
rate-pressure product (mmHg·bpm)	23983±1293	22915±965	0.19	20237±2394	20541±2574	0.77
maximal heart rate (bpm)	120±4	121±4	0.95	104±7	102±8	0.64

4.3.4 CMR

Patients of the control group underwent no CMR at week 8. No change of the LVEF was demonstrated in response to ECP. At baseline, LVEF was 62±1.6% and post-ECP was 64±1.5% (p=0.2). No significant difference was seen between the baseline and week 8 for the other parameters (see Table 4-8).

Table 4-8: CMR data of the ECP group			
	baseline	week 8	p-value
EF (%)	62±1.6	64±1.5	0.2
ED volume (ml)	151±21	156±25	0.53
LV mass ED (g)	89±24	89±16	0.52
Stroke volume (ml)	94±11	98±14	0.26
Cardiac output (l/min)	6.4±0.8	6.5±1	0.69

4.3.5 Invasive measurements

In the ECP-group, the CFIp increased from 0.08±0.01 to 0.15±0.02 ($p<0.001$), whereas the control-group showed no variation in the index (0.15±0.03 to 0.14±0.02, p=0.7), demonstrating the growth of collateral arteries only in patients who were treated with ECP (Figure 4-9). In accordance with the CFIp, the FFR-index increased in the ECP-group from 0.68±0.03 to 0.79±0.03 (p=0.001), but not in the control-group (0.68±0.06 to 0.70±0.05, p=0.4, Figure 4-10). It was necessary to exclude 2/16 patients in the ECP-group and 1/7 in the control-group from analysis after completion of the trial due to protocol violations (ECP) and an arteriovenous-fistula in the ROI (control). However, the number needed to treat (n=12 and n=6) was maintained. The treatment-related effect of ECP remained significant, albeit all data (plus excluded patients) was analyzed (n=16, p=0.018 and p=0.004 for the change of CFIp and FFR accordingly). The severity of the stenosis, as it is angiographically assessed, remained unchanged in both groups during the seven-week period.

The mean variability of Tmn under hyperemia within a set of 3 measurements was 7.6±3.2% at baseline and 6.6±4.8% at follow-up (p=ns). It did not differ between the groups at any time. The IMRcor. remained unchanged in both groups from week 0 to week 8 suggesting no effect of the ECP therapy on the coronary microcirculation. Furthermore, we found that the IMR is always overestimated when the collateral blood flow is not taken into account. At week 0, IMRcor.=12.9±1.8mmHg•sec (or U) and IMR=14.8±2.0U differ significantly (p=<0.001). The same was observed at week 8: IMRcor.=13.7±1.1U and IMR=16.6±1.2U (p=0.001). On the other hand, the central venous pressure does not seem to contribute significantly to the calculation of the IMR. IMRcvp at baseline was 12.9±1.8U and at week 8 it was 13.4±1U. Both values did not differ from the IMRcor.

Females achieved higher FFR values than did males at week 8, although there was no difference in the values at baseline. In particular, at week 8, females had a mean FFR=0.87±0.03 and males had a mean FFR=0.73±0.04 (p=0.04). No change in the CFIp was seen between the two genders. The ΔFFR tended also to differ between the groups (p=0.06) with females having a greater improvement in FFR from week 0 to week 8.

In both groups, no difference of the invasive endpoints was found in relation to other baseline factors (Table 4-9).

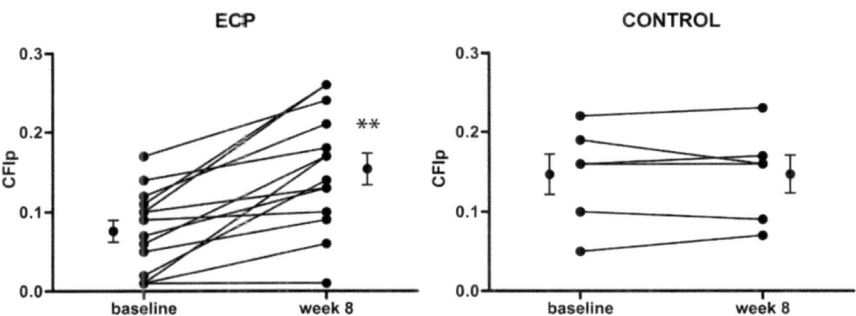

Figure 4.9: *Changes of the CFIp from baseline to week 8, **p<0.001*

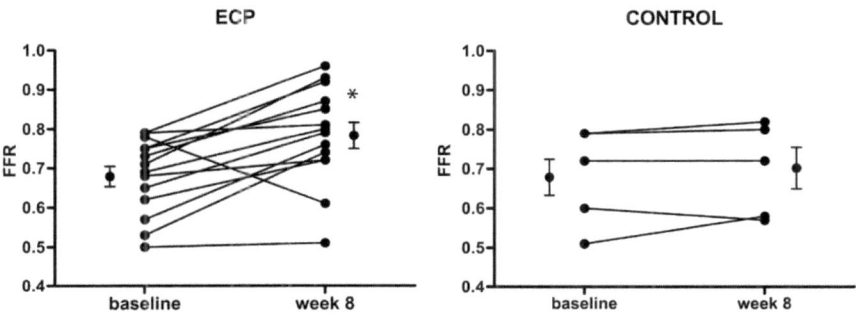

Figure 4.10: *Changes of the FFR from baseline to week 8, * p=0.001*

Table 4-9: Hemodynamic results						
	ECP			Control		
	baseline	week 8	p-value	baseline	week 8	p-value
Systolic BP, mmHg	121.9±2.8	120.4±2.8	0.53	120±7.1	124±3.4	0.52
Diastolic BP, mmHg	70.4±1.76	69.7±1.85	0.45	72±3.44	74±3.08	0.22
CFIp, no unit	0.08±0.01	0.15±0.02	< 0.001*	0.15±0.03	0.14±0.02	0.67
FFR, no unit	0.68±0.03	0.79±0.03	0.001†	0.68±0.05	0.70±0.05	0.39
IMRcor, mmHg • sec	14.2±2.47	15.2±1.43	0.76	10.1±2.48	12±0.86	0.49
Tmn, sec	0.28±0.05	0.28±0.04	0.98	0.21±0.04	0.34±0.08	0.25
Pa, mmHg	80.9±4.1	81.1±4.8	0.96	80.6±3.2	79±9.4	0.87
Pd, mmHg	55.4±2.4	63.1±3.8	0.049†	55.8±4.9	56.8±9.3	0.9
Pw, mmHg	10.2±1.4	18.6±2.3	<0.001*	17±2.8	19.2±2.7	0.31
LVEDP, mmHg	11.6±0.72	11±0.54	0.24	13.5±1.5	12.5±1.18	0.31
Diameter stenosis (%)	52.4±3.46	49.9±4.42	0.22	54.2±4.3	55.0±4.66	0.29

*$p<0.001$, †$p<0.05$. BP=blood pressure, CFIp=pressure derived collateral flow index, ECP=external counterpulsation,
FFR=fractional flow reserve, IMRcor=index of microvascular resistance corrected for the Pw, LVEDP=left ventricular end-diastolic pressure, Tmn=hyperemic transit mean time, Pa=aortic pressure under maximal vasodilatation, Pd=distal coronary pressure under maximal vasodilatation, Pw=coronary occlusive pressure

The presence of symptoms at baseline was a predictor of the response to ECP therapy. Seven patients had no angina at baseline. In this group, FFR did not change significantly (FFR per vs. post-ECP, p=0.19). CFIp increased in this group from 0.08±0.02 to 0.16±0.03 (p=0.014). However, the rest of the seven patients who had angina at baseline showed as a group a highly significant change in the FFR (p=0.001) and CFIp (p=0.008) from baseline to week 8. As in the case of angina, only patients who had dyspnea at the baseline had an improvement in the FFR (p=0.01) and CFIp (p=0.05) after ECP (see Figures 4-11 and 4-12).

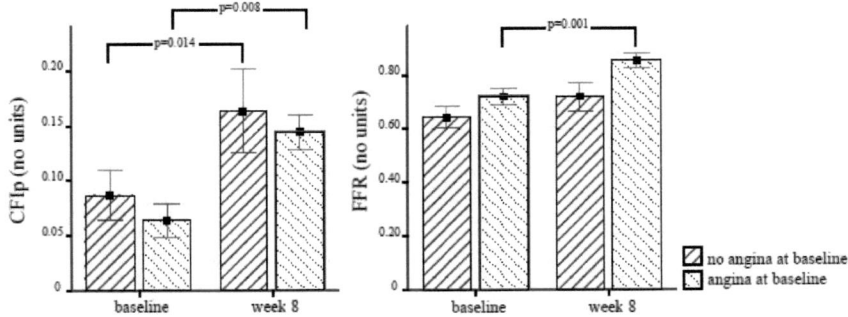

Figure 4-11: *CFIp and FFR changes in relation to angina at the baseline*

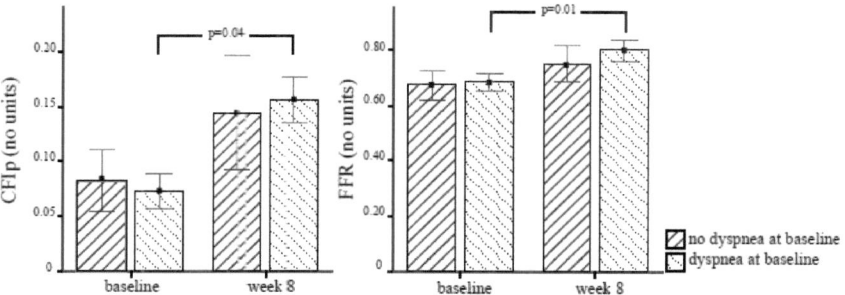

Figure 4-12: *CFIp and FFR changes in relation to dyspnea at exertion at the baseline*

4.3.6 Univariate analysis

A predictor of a positive answer to the therapy was the active way of life. Patients who were doing any kind of exercise on a regular basis prior to study-inclusion (n=8) and who continued this way of life throughout the therapy had greater collateral artery growth and improvement of blood flow than sedentary patients of the ECP group. The mean increase in CFIp for patients with an active way of life was 0.09±0.02, but only 0.01±0.03 (p=0.03) in the sedentary group. Figure 4-13 shows the relative changes of in CFIp for patients who had an active way of life in comparison to sedentary patients.

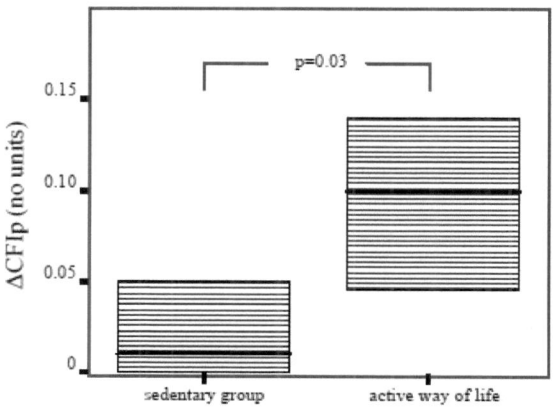

Figure 4-13: *ΔCFIp in relation to the physical way of life*

5 Discussion

Important hallmarks of arteriogenesis are enhanced levels of shear stress across recruited collateral pathways. Experimentally, a therapeutic increase in shear stress may be achieved by artificial stenosis, ligation or arterio-venous shunting distal the site of occlusion/stenosis [38]. ECP increases arterial shear stress even in the absence of a stenosis [172]. In humans, it is proposed as an elegant method to enhance non-invasively the shear stress in the arterial system (within the cardiac diastole without increasing heart rate) [100, 173]. In this proof-of-concept trial, we evaluated whether counterpulsation leads to a significant change in collateral flow index (CFIp) and fractional flow reserve (FFR) in comparison to the natural course under optimal medical treatment. We further investigated whether the clinical improvement of patients correlates with an improvement in myocardial perfusion.

5.1 Establishment and feasibility of the therapy

The external counterpulsation therapy was established in the Franz-Volhard Klinik as a unique non-invasive method for the treatment of patients with stable angina. To our knowledge, only two centers in Germany currently offer the ECP therapy, although a series of data support its effectiveness and safety. The reasons for an inadequate use of the method are that the equipment is expensive, there is a lack of insurance coverage for the therapy, and there is a need for a separate room and for educated operators and supervision by a medical doctor.

Since ECP is largely unknown in Europe, it was very important – prior to the initiation of the study- to update the cardiologists and ambulant offices involved about ECP and the clinical findings that support its effectiveness. Patients with CAD who were appropriate for study inclusion and their family doctors/cardiologists were informed in detail about the therapy. Patients who were interested had a test ECP treatment of 30 minutes to get to know the therapy and to ensure that they could tolerate the treatment. The majority of the patients reported a positive feeling after the test, like that experienced after an endurance run and provided positive feedback to the referring physicians. No patient withdrew after being recruited in the study protocol.

5.2 Clinical benefit of ECP

The present study confirmed the results of previous trials that external counterpulsation improves subjectively the angina symptoms of the patients. Most of the patients in the active group reported an improvement in angina severity of more than 50% after ECP when compared to the severity at baseline. Furthermore, only patients in the ECP group reported an improved exercise capacity after ECP, although this could not be quantified in the exercise test. Most of the previous trials have shown a reduction of at least one class of the CCS classification in more than 70% of the patients who have been treated with ECP [97, 112, 119, 120, 122, 124]. The MUST-trial, a randomized, sham-controlled, double-blind, ECP-trial demonstrated that patients who completed 34 hours of active ECP therapy had a significant reduction in the number of daily episodes of angina in comparison to the ECP-sham group [83].

In the Art.Net.2 trial, the observed reduction of angina and dyspnea at exercise from baseline to post-ECP is in accordance with data from previous trials. These data confirm that ECP is an effective treatment for angina leading either to complete relief from angina (CCS 0) or to an increase of the threshold at which the symptoms appear (reduction of CCS).

The clinical improvement seen in all of the initial symptomatic patients in response to the therapy was correlated with the improvement of the fractional flow reserve and the collateral growth. These data suggest that the clinical improvement within the study-group is mainly a result of the improvement of coronary blood flow and especially of the collateral flow. Other factors, like an improved endothelial function, may also contribute to the clinical benefit as reported by other investigators, although they were not tested in our trial [85, 112, 113].

As mentioned previously in Chapter 4.3.5, only patients with angina or dyspnea at baseline showed a significant increase in both CFIp and FFR. This fact strengthens the hypothesis that the presence of symptoms at baseline is a predictor of a response to ECP. On the other hand, all patients who showed no response to the therapy (no improvement in CFIp or FFR) were asymptomatic at baseline. One could hypothesize that symptomatic patients have a more severe ischemia and, at the same time, a stronger pro-arteriogenic stimulus than patients with no symptoms. The correlation between severity of the angina at baseline and clinical outcome at the end of the therapy has been already demonstrated by other trials. Data from the IEPR (international enhanced external counterpulsation patients registry) suggest that severe angina at baseline (CCS $\geq$ III) is associated with an immediate, favorable response to the therapy [84, 174]. However, we did not find a correlation between the hemodynamic severity of the stenosis (FFR value) at baseline and clinical improvement after ECP.

It is interesting to note that the improvement of dyspnea at exercise was seen to be independent of an increase in the CFIp or FFR. In the absence of an increase in the myocardial perfusion and collateral growth, the latter beneficial effect of ECP may be a result of other effects of the therapy. As mentioned in Chapter 1.3.3, these effects include improvement of the endothelial function and a reduction of the peripheral resistance. Previous trials have, indeed, demonstrated clinical benefits for the patients (reduction of angina) in the absence of an improvement of primary end points like myocardial perfusion [85] or cardiac wall abnormalities [124].

Although the number of patients was small, we did find some difference in the effect of ECP on males and females. At baseline, the prevalence of angina was higher among females than males, although there was no difference in the functional stenosis severity in relation to the gender (FFR=0.66 ± 0.03 in males and FFR=0.71 ± 0.03 in females, p=ns). A higher prevalence of angina among females has been described in large epidemiological studies, even if the severity of angina is adjusted for age or the applied diagnostics and therapy [175]. The causes of angina in women may be broader and involve more factors than those in the solely obstructive coronary artery disease. Alterations of the vascular structure (e.g., stiffness) or the functional capacity of the vessels (e.g., reduced reactivity due to endothelial dysfunction) occur more often in females than they do in males [176]. Angina may occur in this case because of epicardial vascular spasm, epicardial coronary endothelial dysfunction and microvascular disease [177]. At the conclusion of the therapy, females had a significantly higher increase in the FFR than males and this finding was in agreement with the clinical outcome. On the other hand, CFIp changes from baseline to post-ECP were not associated with the gender. So, the higher increase in FFR in women may be associated, as previously mentioned, to the more severe angina of this group at baseline and is not necessarily a gender-associated response to the ECP. However, trials with a larger number of patients could investigate this result.

It is also interesting to note that our data does not support a shortening of the therapy. Throughout the course of ECP, there was a progressive decrease in the number of angina symptoms. However, the improvement in both CCS and NYHA classes was significant only at the end of the therapy. This suggests that the commonly used ECP protocol of 35 single therapies is indeed necessary for an adequate clinical response. It is known that the growth of collateral arteries in humans, contrary to those in animals, is a process that takes place during a longer period of time, from several weeks to months [31].

In summary, the improvement of angina in the current trial was closely associated with an improvement in the myocardial and collateral blood flow.

5.3 Exercise test and ECP

No significant changes of any parameters of the exercise test were found in the ECP group. Whether ECP improves exercise duration or the ischemic threshold of the patients remains unclear, as previous results have produced controversial results. Novo et al showed an improvement in exercise capacity at the cycloergometer (increase in exercise time of 21%) without a change in the ischemic threshold [124]. In accordance with these results, Michaels et al showed an improvement in exercise time and angina-free time that was not accompanied by a reduction of perfusion defects by scintigraphy [85].

On the other hand, a correlation of reduction of ischemic defects and improvement in the exercise duration was shown by Tartaglia [87]. Of interest is that the MUST study [83] also demonstrated an increase in the time to >1mm ST-segment depression in the active ECP group, in comparison to the sham group, implying an improvement of exercise-induced ischemia. No significant difference in the duration of the exercise between the groups was found. Furthermore, Masuda and colleagues [109] demonstrated an improvement in myocardial perfusion, despite an absence of any significant change in exercise duration or double product.

We observed no effect of ECP on parameters of the ergometric test. A possible reason for this, aside from the low number of patients, might have been the high percentage of patients on β-blocker (100%) that may lead to a fixed exercise duration [178]. The intake of β-blockers was much higher in the current study than in all previous trials of ECP (intake of 63%-83%). It is interesting to note that the patients in our trial had, in comparison to previous trials with similar exercise protocols, longer exercise durations at baseline. The mean exercise duration at baseline was 416±28s, while in the previous trials, the pre-ECP duration was always below 400s [86, 87, 122, 124, 125]. This may be associated with the high prevalence of angina-free patients at baseline in the current trial (56%) and the high compliance to the prescribed medication. The most common cause for the early cessation of the exercise tests, either at baseline or at week 8, was muscular exhaustion or orthopedic complaints and not angina. In this case, the observed clinical improvement at week 8 may not contribute to a prolongation of exercise duration. Furthermore, there was a low use of nitrates by our patients (28%) in comparison to an intake of 88%-100% in the studies that showed an improvement in exercise duration [85, 87, 125]. Nitroglycerine is related to a preconditioning effect that improves the outcome of exercise tests, including prolonged exercise duration and ischemic threshold [179, 180].

In conclusion, this clinical endpoint is of limited value due to the cessation of the test by more than 50% of the patients due to muscular exhaustion or orthopedic complaints.

5.4 ECP, arteriogenesis and myocardial blood flow

5.4.1 Stimulation of arteriogenesis by ECP

The Art.Net.2 trial demonstrated for the first time the improvement of the myocardial collateral network by invasive hemodynamic measurements in response to external counterpulsation therapy. The collateral blood-flow was assessed by the pressure-related collateral flow index (CFIp). The CFIp is currently the gold standard for the assessment of collateral circulation and was used as the primary endpoint within our trial.

CFIp expresses the collateral blood flow maintained during coronary occlusion relative to normal antegrade flow during vessel patency [59]. The significant increases of the collateral blood flow and myocardial blood flow in response to external counterpulsation are the major results of this trial. Patients with stable coronary artery disease and at least one significant residual stenosis can improve their collateral arteries and receive a clinical benefit in response to this "passive training." In other words, counterpulsation has the potential to trigger coronary arteriogenesis and improve the blunted myocardial blood flow due to the presence of an epicardial stenosis. The significant increase of CFIp (0.07 ± 0.016) in our study - however moderate - is explained by the heterogeneity of patients with moderate to severe stenosis. As explained below, patients with more severe stenoses could lead to a greater increase in the CFIp index. However, patients with severe coronary artery stenosis, who are known to be at a higher risk of periprocedural complications [135], had to be excluded from this longitudinal trial due to ethical concerns. The close correlation of the degree of stenosis and the conductance of collaterals (CFIp) is in accordance with earlier experimental data in this field by Schaper [181], as well as with several clinical trials [39, 47]. Although the functional severity of the stenosis and symptoms at baseline were well matched, collateral blood flow differed between the two study groups of our trial, reflecting the high inter-individual range of the collateral status. These inter-individual variations are well known in CAD patients – as previously published [39, 47, 67, 73] and provoked in patients with poor collateralization (CFIp < 0.25). All patients in our trial had insufficient collateralization at baseline and showed a significant increase in collateral blood flow only after ECP treatment. The CFIp index at baseline was slightly lower in our study compared to previous trials (mean CFIp = 0.13 ± 0.1) [39]. The low CFIp values in our study may be interpreted to mean that the residual stenoses were not as highly relevant as indicated from the mean percent diameter stenosis of all included patients, which was $53\pm2.3\%$. The percent diameter stenosis is the only multivariate predictor of functional important collateral blood flow. Pohl and colleagues demonstrated that patients with poor collaterals (CFIp<0.25) had a percent diameter stenosis of $76\pm14\%$ and patients with good collaterals (CFIp>0.25) had a mean percent diameter stenosis of $82\pm15\%$ [39]. Taking into account the fact, that in our study the mean percent of diameter stenosis at baseline of 53% was relatively low, it is reasonable to argue that despite the improvement of the CFIp in 85% of the patients, only two of them had good collaterals post-ECP. Since the publication of the data of the Art.Net.2 Trial [182, 183], another clinical study in the field of ECP and collateral artery growth was published [184]. In the latter trial, a very similar study protocol was used to assess a possible arteriogenic effect of ECP. The results of this trial verified our results and provide one more piece of evidence to justify the stimulation of collateral growth by external counterpulsation. Patients were divided into a group undergoing ECP at cuff pressures of 300 mm Hg and a sham-group receiving ECP therapy at cuff pressures of 80 mm Hg. After 30 h of therapy, the CFIp increased in the active group from 0.12 to 0.17, but not in the sham-group. In accordance with our results, the FFR also improved from 0.85 to 0.91. An increase of the FFR, independent of the baseline values, was common in both trials. In the study by Gloekler et al, the patients had an FFR>0.8 at baseline, despite angiographic severe stenoses of about 65%. In our trial, patients had hemodynamic severe stenoses (FFR<0.8) in the presence of moderate angiographic stenoses. The fact that each study had patients with either angiographic or hemodynamic severe stenoses may have led to the moderate increase of CFIp that was seen in both trials.

5.4.2 ECP compared to pharmacologic stimulation of arteriogenesis

Beside the biomechanical pro-arteriogenic effect observed in the aforementioned ECP trials, pharmacologic stimulation of arteriogenesis is also possible. The effect of application of GM-

CSF in inducing arteriogenesis by invasive pressure measurements has been tested [67]. GM-CSF is a strong arteriogenic peptide that results in an increased number and diameter of collateral arteries [185, 186]. Seiler and colleagues showed that treatment with GM-CSF over a period of 14 days leads to a significant improvement of CFIp in comparison to a placebo group. In this trial, the mean percent of diameter stenosis at baseline was 71%±12 and the mean CFIp=0.21±0.14. At the end of the study period, CFIp increased to 0.31±0.23 [67]. However, due to the differing degree of stenosis and the period of treatment (2 weeks GM-CSF vs. 7 weeks ECP), no conclusion can be drawn about the effectiveness of either treatment (GM-CSF vs. ECP).

5.4.3 Collateral and myocardial blood flow

The second endpoint in our trial, the fractional flow reserve (FFR), increased significantly after ECP. The FFR is an index that takes into account the contribution of collaterals, as long as the distal coronary pressure during maximal hyperemia reflects both antegrade and retrograde flow [151]. The parallel improvement of the CFIp and FFR in angiographically unchanged coronary arteries provides evidence that the proliferation of the collateral arteries contribute to the improved myocardial blood flow that leads to the clinical improvement of the patient. The contribution of the collateral arteries, as reflected in the FFR index, may be further strengthened by the fact that the microcirculation (assessed by the IMR index) remained unchanged in response to ECP. If an alteration of the distal microvascular resistance had occurred, the adenosine-induced dilatation and, therefore, the distal pressure and the FFR value could have been influenced. In this case, a change of the FFR would, at least in part, reflect a change of the cardiac microcirculation and not only of the collateral flow. However, we did not find any change of microcirculatory resistance in our trial.

Furthermore, the quantitative angiography did not show any change in stenosis severity during the trial (8 weeks). This supports further our data suggesting that the increase of the FFR reflects the 'true' improvement of myocardial blood flow and is not based on changes in the degree of stenosis or microvascular resistance.

It is also worth mentioning that the FFR is not only an index of the trans-stenotic pressure loss due to a stenosis. It is calculated as the ratio of distal to aortic pressure under maximal hyperemia (when epicardial and microvascular resistance are minimal) and thus also reflects myocardial perfusion. Consequently, an improvement of the FFR in response to ECP represents an improvement of the blood flow to the part of the myocardium that is supplied by the narrowed artery [161].

5.4.4 Clinical impact of ECP treatment

All study participants were qualified for PCI at baseline due to pathological FFR (FFR<0.8) and positive ischemic testing [21]. At the end of the 7-week therapy course 6/16 patients in the ECP-group versus 1/7 patients in the control-group were deferred from angioplasty since the FFR had improved to levels above 0.8 accompanied by a reduction, or even complete relief of angina. So, these patients had no reason to undergo PCI after the ECP treatment, despite being candidates for PCI treatment before inclusion in the study protocol.

5.4.5 New data on the mechanism of action of ECP

In summary, our data suggest the improvement of the myocardial flow reserve after ECP, reflecting at the same time an improved myocardial blood flow in the area at risk. Most of the previous trials have used non-invasive techniques to investigate the effect of ECP on myocardial ischemia. By N-ammonia positron emission tomography, Masuda and colleagues showed an improvement of myocardial perfusion after therapy in the regions of stenotic vessels [109]. Other research groups, by performing myocardial scintigraphy combined with exercise tests have demonstrated a reduction of the perfusion defects after ECP correlated to reduced anginal symptoms [86, 87, 120, 122].

Until our trial, only one study had used invasive methods to assess the effect of ECP on the cardiac collateral vessels and had shown no improvement of the angiographic Rentrop score after ECP [86]. The latter method is, however, less sensitive and observer-dependent than the pressure-derived collateral flow index.

However, as mentioned previously, other trials showed no effect of ECP on the myocardial ischemia. They suggested the peripheral ("training") effect of the therapy and an improved endothelial function as a mechanism to explain the subjective improvement of the patients' symptoms [85, 110]. As mentioned above (Chapter 1.3.3.2), a weakness of the previous studies was that the exercise stress test was performed at the same level pre- and post-ECP. In this case, a reduced myocardial oxygen demand due to lower peripheral resistance could also explain the attenuation of perfusion defects and the relief of the patients' symptoms. In our trial, myocardial blood flow was assessed at each point in time by FFR under maximal vasodilatation (and maximal hyperemia) induced by intravenous injection of adenosine. Under maximal vasodilatation, the vascular resistance is minimal and assumed to be constant. So, in each invasive measurement, we assessed changes of the myocardial blood flow under maximal stress and not at a pre-defined level of stress (or exercise). In this case, structural or functional changes of the coronary vasculature during the seven weeks may be translated to increases of myocardial flow under the maximal action of adenosine. Furthermore, measurements of FFR under maximal hyperemia assure reproducible results, independently of the systemic hemodynamic [153].

Although we showed a clear effect of ECP on coronary collateral growth, other factors may also contribute to the mechanism of action of ECP. As mentioned in Chapter 1.3.3, the mechanism of action of ECP is complex. The hypothesis that counterpulsation improves the endothelial function was confirmed by measurements of the peripheral endothelial function by several different investigators. The main findings were that an improvement of the peripheral endothelial function correlates with the decrease of the CCS classes [112, 113]. Recently, it was confirmed that the improvement of the CFIp correlates with the improvement of the peripheral endothelial function assessed by flow mediated dilation [184]. Whether the coronary endothelial function is also improved after ECP or not has not been directly investigated. However, data from the literature indicate that peripheral and coronary endothelial functions correlate well with each other [187]. In this case, ECP would improve angina not only by reducing peripheral resistance and the myocardial oxygen demand, but also by leading to improved vasodilation of the epicardial coronary arteries and thus to improved myocardial perfusion.

In the bibliography, there are a few case reports about the effect of ECP on the coronary endothelial function. Bonetti and colleagues reported a case of a patient with symptomatic coronary endothelial dysfunction in the absence of obstructive coronary disease who was successful treated with ECP [128]. ECP led to complete relief of angina. In another report, a series of patients with syndrome X and a positive stress test demonstrating myocardial ischemia at baseline were treated with ECP. All patients had an improvement of clinical symptoms and 93% of them had no ischemic defects at the final imaging stress test [127]. These results are compatible with previous findings from a trial that assessed the effect of four weeks of exercise training in patients who had impaired coronary endothelial functions. It was demonstrated that the endothelium-dependent (assessed by injection of acetylcholine) coronary vasodilatation increased after training [188]. As long as exercise and ECP share common vascular effects, like an increase of shear stress in the vascular system, it is reasonable to assume that ECP also exerts effects on coronary endothelium.

The attenuation of the endothelial dysfunction after ECP that has been seen in previous trials could explain the clinical improvement of the patients even if no direct cardiac effects occur. In response to increased shear stress, ECP leads to a release of nitric oxide, peripheral vasodilatation and a reduction of the resistance/arterial stiffness. Consequently, cardiac afterload and myocardial oxygen demand are reduced, leading to relief of angina symptoms. This mechanism of action has been proposed by performing applanation tonometry of the radial artery before and after a course of ECP [117]. However, other investigators who used the same method did not show any change of arterial stiffness [125].

In summary, the present data support a multifactor mechanism of ECP, including at least collateral artery growth and improved endothelial function.

5.4.6 Effectiveness ratio and response to the therapy

The effectiveness or the diastolic to systolic ratio (D/S ratio) is used to estimate the hemodynamic changes occurring during the ECP. Most of the previous trials have suggested a direct relation of an improvement of the ratio to a clinical improvement of the patient. Previous data from 2,486 patients treated with ECP have identified the D/S ratio at baseline and its relative change after the therapy as a predictor of the clinical response to ECP. A D/S ratio ≤0.7 at baseline is generally characterized as low, whereas a D/S >0.7 is considered to be high. Patients, who initially had low D.S ratios and high D/S ratios at the end of ECP, benefited more from the ECP therapy. Independent predictors of a high D/S ratio at baseline include the male gender, an age <65, an absence of non-cardiac vascular disease, smoking, hypertension, heart failure, diabetes mellitus and previous CABG surgery [96]. Other investigators have suggested that a D/S ratio >1.5 is associated with improved short and long term clinical outcomes [95]. On the other hand, another trial, although confirming gender and age as predictors of the baseline D/S ratio, showed that the benefit from the therapy is independent of a change in the index during the therapy [97]. The main finding in our study is that the improvement of angina and the invasive parameters correlate with an improvement in the D/S ratio. The improvement in the D/S ratio mirrors a decrease of arterial stiffness that can be attributed, in part, to attenuation of endothelial dysfunction [189]. The latter is supported by previous trials as mentioned above (see Chapter 1.3.3.2).

5.5 Effect on coronary microcirculation

Microvascular dysfunction in the presence of obstructive coronary artery disease not only reflects an attenuated endothelial dependent vasodilatation as a result of traditional coronary risk factors (diabetes, hypertension, smoking, hyperlipidemia, and insulin-resistance). It may induce constriction of the distal pre-arterioles and arterioles or inadequate subepicardial pre-arteriolar dilatation, causing myocardial ischemia that is not necessarily related to the degree of epicardial stenosis [157, 190]. We assessed the effect of ECP on the coronary microvasculature by using the index of microcirculatory resistance (IMR). This index demonstrates the ability of the microcirculation to dilate in response to a vasodilator agent (like adenosine) causing an increase of myocardial blood flow. The IMR at baseline and the IMR after ECP did not differ significantly and showed an unchanged microvascular resistance. This means that ECP probably has no effect on the microcirculation when this is assessed at maximal hyperemia by infusion of adenosine. As long as adenosine primarily reflects an endothelium-independent vasodilatation, one cannot exclude a possible effect of ECP on the endothelium-dependent vasodilatation as mentioned above (see Chapter 5.4.5). This was the first study to assess the effect of ECP on microvascular resistance. Although there is no cut-off value for the index, an IMR=22mmHg•sec (or U) was found in a previous trial in patients without obvious microvascular dysfunction and without diabetes, possibly suggesting a normal value [162]. In our study the mean IMR=12.9U at baseline revealed a normal myocardial microvascular function in these patients. An improvement of the already normal microvascular function should not be expected after ECP.

5.5.1 Hemodynamic aspects of IMR

In the current trial we evaluated for the first time in patients who had chronic coronary stenoses the hypothesis that an additional measurement of the coronary occlusion pressure is necessary to calculate the index of microcirculatory resistance. We demonstrated that to accurately assess the IMR, it is necessary to measure the actual coronary occlusion pressure (Pw). When IMR is calculated only on the basis of transit mean time and distal pressure, it will be overestimated, regardless of whether the epicardial stenosis is severe (FFR<0.75) or not (FFR≥0.75). Previous data suggested that in moderate to severe epicardial stenoses (0.52<FFR<0.69), the IMR increases with increasing stenosis severity, whereas the IMRcor.

remains stable [162]. Our data, in patients with chronic moderate to mild stenoses (mean FFR at baseline=0.69, mean FFR at follow-up=0.76) indicate that this overestimation is independent of the severity of the stenosis. A major challenge of our invasive protocol was that Pw was measured during both catheterizations at the end of a 60s balloon occlusion, as indicated for correct assessment of the collateral status [60]. Consequently, the actual values of Pw, Pd and Pa were used to calculate the IMRcor at the two different times. In contrast, in previous trials the Pw was measured only one time [162]. Thereafter, the IMRcor. was calculated upon this unique Pw value together with different values of Pd and Pa, which were obtained under different degrees of coronary stenoses. So, in the current trial, the influence of the coronary stenosis on IMR was assessed by taking into account the actual collateral status for each functional stenosis severity.

Another important aspect of the current trial is that we conducted the two invasive measurements in the absence of any coronary intervention between these points in time. This minimizes a possible change of the microcirculatory resistance due to vasoconstriction or distal embolization caused by a percutaneous intervention [191, 192]. We demonstrated that IMR can be used for intra-individual measurements in studies performing a follow-up catheterization in a period of a few weeks. Thus, IMR, when measured properly, is a reproducible index, independent of the hemodynamic status of the patient as it was previously shown under different hemodynamic conditions during a single catheterization procedure [193].

5.6 Effect of ECP on the left ventricular function

By using cardiac magnetic resonance, we found that ECP does not influence the left ventricular systolic function. All patients in the ECP group had a normal ejection fraction (EF) at baseline that remained statistically unchanged following the treatment period. CMR is suggested as the gold standard method for evaluation of the left ventricular function [194, 195]. Our results are in accordance with a recently published trial that indicated no effect of ECP on different echocardiographic parameters of the left ventricular systolic and diastolic function, despite clinical improvement of the patients [132]. It is also reported that patients with EF <50% at baseline do not have any additional benefit of the EF after ECP [131]. However, in a previous trial that included patients who had heart failure, LVEF increased from 40% to 46% [196]. So, for patients with a stable coronary artery disease and a normal left ventricular ejection fraction, changes of the EF or other characteristics of the left ventricle may not play a role in the clinical improvement following ECP.

5.7 Limitations of the study

The limitations of this study are a) the lack of a sham group and b) the delayed recruitment of the control group. With regards to the first limitation, the local ethical committee did not approve treating patients with sham treatments. In previous trials, a low cuff pressure of 75-80 mm of Hg was used as a sham counterpulsation therapy. All previous trials, including a sham group, have demonstrated significant changes of the end points only in the groups that received active counterpulsation therapy. The MUST-trial showed a significant benefit of the active therapy (cuff pressure 300 mm Hg) in regard to clinical end points (angina episodes, use of nitroglycerine) compared to the sham group (cuff pressure 75 mm Hg) [83]. Levenson et al showed that active counterpulsation is more effective in reducing carotid stiffness and vascular resistance in patients with coronary artery disease [197]. In another study by the same investigators, it was demonstrated that one hour of sham-ECP does not have any effect on the release of cGMP when compared to active therapy [114]. In the trial by Goekler et al, which is similar to our own, the sham group did not show any statistically significant changes in the FFR or the CFIp index as did the active ECP group [184]. Furthermore, previous data suggest that a change in the CFIp within two to three months, in the absence of any coronary intervention or modification of the medical treatment, is not to be expected. It was reported that it is, instead, a trend towards a decrease in the index when two invasive pressure measurements are sequentially performed within three months [39]. Despite all previous data that suggest that the clinical benefit of ECP is related only to the active therapy [83], a placebo effect cannot be excluded. In the case of ECP, this effect may be considerable, since it is known that therapies that involve medical devices can be associated with an enhanced placebo effect [198].

To compensate for the lack of a sham group, we applied for a control-group, receiving optimal medication and counseling as performed in COURAGE. The positive vote for this control was obtained after the trial was initiated. Hence, a "regular" randomization with the start of the trial was not feasible.

6 References

1. Destatis. *Todesursachen- und Bevölkerungsstatistiken*. 2009 [Available from: http://www.destatis.de/jetspeed/portal/cms/.
2. F. van Buuren, D.H., *23. Bericht über die Leistungszahlen der Herzkatheterlabore in der Bundesrepublik Deutschland*. Kardiologe 2009(3): p. 437–442.
3. Gummert, J.F., A. Funkat, A. Beckmann, et al., *Cardiac surgery in Germany during 2008. A report on behalf of the German Society for Thoracic and Cardiovascular Surgery*. Thorac Cardiovasc Surg, 2009. **57**(6): p. 315-23.
4. Forster, T. *Krankheitskostenrechnung für Deutschland* 2004 [cited; Available from: http://www.destatis.de.
5. Rader, D.J. and A. Daugherty, *Translating molecular discoveries into new therapies for atherosclerosis*. Nature, 2008. **451**(7181): p. 904-13.
6. Bassand, J.P., C.W. Hamm, D. Ardissino, et al., *Guidelines for the diagnosis and treatment of non-ST-segment elevation acute coronary syndromes*. Eur Heart J, 2007. **28**(13): p. 1598-660.
7. Fox, K., M.A. Garcia, D. Ardissino, et al., *Guidelines on the management of stable angina pectoris: executive summary: the Task Force on the Management of Stable Angina Pectoris of the European Society of Cardiology*. Eur Heart J, 2006. **27**(11): p. 1341-81.
8. Schinkel, A.F., J.J. Bax, M.L. Geleijnse, et al., *Noninvasive evaluation of ischaemic heart disease: myocardial perfusion imaging or stress echocardiography?* Eur Heart J, 2003. **24**(9): p. 789-800.
9. Lodge, M.A., H. Braess, F. Mahmoud, et al., *Developments in nuclear cardiology: transition from single photon emission computed tomography to positron emission tomography-computed tomography*. J Invasive Cardiol, 2005. **17**(9): p. 491-6.
10. Al-Saadi, N., E. Nagel, M. Gross, et al., *Noninvasive detection of myocardial ischemia from perfusion reserve based on cardiovascular magnetic resonance*. Circulation, 2000. **101**(12): p. 1379-83.
11. Jahnke, C., E. Nagel, R. Gebker, et al., *Prognostic value of cardiac magnetic resonance stress tests: adenosine stress perfusion and dobutamine stress wall motion imaging*. Circulation, 2007. **115**(13): p. 1769-76.
12. Weustink, A.C., N.R. Mollet, L.A. Neefjes, et al., *Diagnostic accuracy and clinical utility of noninvasive testing for coronary artery disease*. Ann Intern Med, 2010. **152**(10): p. 630-9.
13. Anderson, K.M., P.M. Odell, P.W. Wilson, and W.B. Kannel, *Cardiovascular disease risk profiles*. Am Heart J, 1991. **121**(1 Pt 2): p. 293-8.
14. Fraker, T.D., Jr., S.D. Fihn, R.J. Gibbons, et al., *2007 chronic angina focused update of the ACC/AHA 2002 guidelines for the management of patients with chronic stable angina: a report of the American College of Cardiology/American Heart Association Task Force on Practice Guidelines Writing Group to develop the focused update of the 2002 guidelines for the management of patients with chronic stable angina*. J Am Coll Cardiol, 2007. **50**(23): p. 2264-74.
15. Cannon, C.P., B.A. Steinberg, S.A. Murphy, J.L. Mega, and E. Braunwald, *Meta-analysis of cardiovascular outcomes trials comparing intensive versus moderate statin therapy*. J Am Coll Cardiol, 2006. **48**(3): p. 438-45.

16. Baigent, C., A. Keech, P.M. Kearney, et al., *Efficacy and safety of cholesterol-lowering treatment: prospective meta-analysis of data from 90,056 participants in 14 randomised trials of statins.* Lancet, 2005. **366**(9493): p. 1267-78.
17. Opie, L.H., P.J. Commerford, and B.J. Gersh, *Controversies in stable coronary artery disease.* The Lancet. **367**(9504): p. 69-78.
18. White, H.D., *Should all patients with coronary disease receive angiotensin-converting-enzyme inhibitors?* The Lancet, 2003. **362**(9386): p. 755-757.
19. Hoffman, S.N., J.A. TenBrook, M.P. Wolf, et al., *A meta-analysis of randomized controlled trials comparing coronary artery bypass graft with percutaneous transluminal coronary angioplasty: one- to eight-year outcomes.* J Am Coll Cardiol, 2003. **41**(8): p. 1293-304.
20. Curtis, J.P. and H.M. Krumholz, *Keeping the patient in view: defining the appropriateness of percutaneous coronary interventions.* Circulation, 2004. **110**(25): p. 3746-8.
21. Silber, S., P. Albertsson, F.F. Aviles, et al., *Guidelines for percutaneous coronary interventions. The Task Force for Percutaneous Coronary Interventions of the European Society of Cardiology.* Eur Heart J, 2005. **26**(8): p. 804-47.
22. Boden, W.E., R.A. O'Rourke, K.K. Teo, et al., *Optimal medical therapy with or without PCI for stable coronary disease.* N Engl J Med, 2007. **356**(15): p. 1503-16.
23. Shaw, L.J., D.S. Berman, D.J. Maron, et al., *Optimal medical therapy with or without percutaneous coronary intervention to reduce ischemic burden: results from the Clinical Outcomes Utilizing Revascularization and Aggressive Drug Evaluation (COURAGE) trial nuclear substudy.* Circulation, 2008. **117**(10): p. 1283-91.
24. Kim, M.C., A. Kini, and S.K. Sharma, *Refractory angina pectoris: mechanism and therapeutic options.* J Am Coll Cardiol, 2002. **39**(6): p. 923-34.
25. Risau, W., *Mechanisms of angiogenesis.* Nature, 1997. **386**(6626): p. 671-4.
26. Ito, W.D., M. Arras, D. Scholz, et al., *Angiogenesis but not collateral growth is associated with ischemia after femoral artery occlusion.* Am J Physiol, 1997. **273**(3 Pt 2): p. H1255-65.
27. Heil, M., I. Eitenmuller, T. Schmitz-Rixen, and W. Schaper, *Arteriogenesis versus angiogenesis: similarities and differences.* J Cell Mol Med, 2006. **10**(1): p. 45-55.
28. Scholz, D., W.J. Cai, and W. Schaper, *Arteriogenesis, a new concept of vascular adaptation in occlusive disease.* Angiogenesis, 2001. **4**(4): p. 247-57.
29. Buschmann, I. and W. Schaper, *Arteriogenesis Versus Angiogenesis: Two Mechanisms of Vessel Growth.* News Physiol Sci, 1999. **14**: p. 121-125.
30. Scholz, D., W. Ito, I. Fleming, et al., *Ultrastructure and molecular histology of rabbit hind-limb collateral artery growth (arteriogenesis).* Virchows Arch, 2000. **436**(3): p. 257-70.
31. William F.M. Fulton, N.v.R., *The coronary collateral circulation in man, in Schaper W., Schaper J. (eds.): Arteriogenesis.* 2004, page 311: Kluwer Academic Publishers. 311.
32. Schaper, W.S.a.J., *Arteriogenesis* 2004: Kluwer Academic Publishers.
33. Cai, W.J., S. Koltai, E. Kocsis, et al., *Remodeling of the adventitia during coronary arteriogenesis.* Am J Physiol Heart Circ Physiol, 2003. **284**(1): p. H31-40.

34. Cai, W.J., E. Kocsis, X. Wu, et al., *Remodeling of the vascular tunica media is essential for development of collateral vessels in the canine heart.* Mol Cell Biochem, 2004. **264**(1-2): p. 201-10.
35. Troidl, C., K. Troidl, W. Schierling, et al., *Trpv4 induces collateral vessel growth during regeneration of the arterial circulation.* J Cell Mol Med, 2008.
36. Demicheva, E., M. Hecker, and T. Korff, *Stretch-Induced Activation of the Transcription Factor Activator Protein-1 Controls Monocyte Chemoattractant Protein-1 Expression During Arteriogenesis.* Circ Res, 2008.
37. Cai, W., R. Vosschulte, A. Afsah-Hedjri, et al., *Altered balance between extracellular proteolysis and antiproteolysis is associated with adaptive coronary arteriogenesis.* J Mol Cell Cardiol, 2000. **32**(6): p. 997-1011.
38. Eitenmuller, I., O. Volger, A. Kluge, et al., *The range of adaptation by collateral vessels after femoral artery occlusion.* Circ Res, 2006. **99**(6): p. 656-62.
39. Pohl, T., C. Seiler, M. Billinger, et al., *Frequency distribution of collateral flow and factors influencing collateral channel development. Functional collateral channel measurement in 450 patients with coronary artery disease.* J Am Coll Cardiol, 2001. **38**(7): p. 1872-8.
40. Schaper, W. and I. Buschmann, *Arteriogenesis, the good and bad of it.* Cardiovasc Res, 1999. **43**(4): p. 835-7.
41. Lee, C.W., S.W. Park, G.Y. Cho, et al., *Pressure-derived fractional collateral blood flow: a primary determinant of left ventricular recovery after reperfused acute myocardial infarction.* J Am Coll Cardiol, 2000. **35**(4): p. 949-55.
42. Hirai, T., M. Fujita, H. Nakajima, et al., *Importance of collateral circulation for prevention of left ventricular aneurysm formation in acute myocardial infarction.* Circulation, 1989. **79**(4): p. 791-6.
43. Ishihara, M., I. Inoue, T. Kawagoe, et al., *Comparison of the cardioprotective effect of prodromal angina pectoris and collateral circulation in patients with a first anterior wall acute myocardial infarction.* Am J Cardiol, 2005. **95**(5): p. 622-5.
44. Nathoe, H.M., J. Koerselman, E. Buskens, et al., *Determinants and prognostic significance of collaterals in patients undergoing coronary revascularization.* Am J Cardiol, 2006. **98**(1): p. 31-5.
45. Hansen, J.F., *Coronary collateral circulation: clinical significance and influence on survival in patients with coronary artery occlusion.* Am Heart J, 1989. **117**(2): p. 290-5.
46. Bruschke, A., *The diagnostic significance of the coronary arteriogram.* 1970: The Netherlands, Utrecht.
47. Meier, P., S. Gloekler, R. Zbinden, et al., *Beneficial effect of recruitable collaterals: a 10-year follow-up study in patients with stable coronary artery disease undergoing quantitative collateral measurements.* Circulation, 2007. **116**(9): p. 975-83.
48. Billinger, M., P. Kloos, F.R. Eberli, et al., *Physiologically assessed coronary collateral flow and adverse cardiac ischemic events. a follow-up study in 403 patients with coronary artery disease.* J Am Coll Cardiol, 2002. **40**(9): p. 1545-50.
49. Hirai, T., M. Fujita, K. Yamanishi, et al., *Significance of preinfarction angina for preservation of left ventricular function in acute myocardial infarction.* Am Heart J, 1992. **124**(1): p. 19-24.

50. Billinger, M., M. Fleisch, F.R. Eberli, et al., *Is the development of myocardial tolerance to repeated ischemia in humans due to preconditioning or to collateral recruitment?* J Am Coll Cardiol, 1999. **33**(4): p. 1027-35.

51. Lambiase, P.D., R.J. Edwards, M.R. Cusack, et al., *Exercise-induced ischemia initiates the second window of protection in humans independent of collateral recruitment.* J Am Coll Cardiol, 2003. **41**(7): p. 1174-82.

52. Nohara, R., H. Kambara, T. Murakami, et al., *Collateral function in early acute myocardial infarction.* Am J Cardiol, 1983. **52**(8): p. 955-9.

53. Seiler, C., *The human coronary collateral circulation.* Heart, 2003. **89**(11): p. 1352-7.

54. Seiler, C., *Function of the Coronary Collateral Circulation in Man, in Schaper W., Schaper J. (eds.): Arteriogenesis.* 2004: Kluster Academic Publishers.

55. Rentrop, K.P., M. Cohen, H. Blanke, and R.A. Phillips, *Changes in collateral channel filling immediately after controlled coronary artery occlusion by an angioplasty balloon in human subjects.* J Am Coll Cardiol, 1985. **5**(3): p. 587-92.

56. Rockstroh, J. and B.G. Brown, *Coronary collateral size, flow capacity, and growth: estimates from the angiogram in patients with obstructive coronary disease.* Circulation, 2002. **105**(2): p. 168-73.

57. Werner, G.S., M. Ferrari, S. Heinke, et al., *Angiographic assessment of collateral connections in comparison with invasively determined collateral function in chronic coronary occlusions.* Circulation, 2003. **107**(15): p. 1972-7.

58. Berry, C., K.P. Balachandran, P.L. L'Allier, et al., *Importance of collateral circulation in coronary heart disease.* Eur Heart J, 2007. **28**(3): p. 278-91.

59. Seiler, C., M. Fleisch, A. Garachemani, and B. Meier, *Coronary collateral quantitation in patients with coronary artery disease using intravascular flow velocity or pressure measurements.* J Am Coll Cardiol, 1998. **32**(5): p. 1272-9.

60. Mason, M.J., D.J. Patel, V. Paul, and C.D. Ilsley, *Time course and extent of collateral channel recruitment during coronary angioplasty.* Coron Artery Dis, 2002. **13**(1): p. 17-23.

61. Pijls, N.H., G.J. Bech, M.I. el Gamal, et al., *Quantification of recruitable coronary collateral blood flow in conscious humans and its potential to predict future ischemic events.* J Am Coll Cardiol, 1995. **25**(7): p. 1522-8.

62. Matsuo, H., S. Watanabe, T. Kadosaki, et al., *Validation of collateral fractional flow reserve by myocardial perfusion imaging.* Circulation, 2002. **105**(9): p. 1060-5.

63. Mohri, M., K. Egashira, T. Kuga, H. Shimokawa, and A. Takeshita, *Correlations between recruitable coronary collateral flow velocities, distal occlusion pressure, and electrocardiographic changes in patients undergoing angioplasty.* Jpn Circ J, 1997. **61**(12): p. 971-8.

64. de Marchi, S.F., P. Oswald, S. Windecker, B. Meier, and C. Seiler, *Reciprocal relationship between left ventricular filling pressure and the recruitable human coronary collateral circulation.* Eur Heart J, 2005. **26**(6): p. 558-66.

65. Doucette, J.W., P.D. Corl, H.M. Payne, et al., *Validation of a Doppler guide wire for intravascular measurement of coronary artery flow velocity.* Circulation, 1992. **85**(5): p. 1899-911.

66. Werner, G.S., E. Jandt, A. Krack, et al., *Growth factors in the collateral circulation of chronic total coronary occlusions: relation to duration of occlusion and collateral function.* Circulation, 2004. **110**(14): p. 1940-5.

67. Seiler, C., T. Pohl, K. Wustmann, et al., *Promotion of collateral growth by granulocyte-macrophage colony-stimulating factor in patients with coronary artery disease: a randomized, double-blind, placebo-controlled study.* Circulation, 2001. **104**(17): p. 2012-7.
68. Hill, J.M., M.A. Syed, A.E. Arai, et al., *Outcomes and risks of granulocyte colony-stimulating factor in patients with coronary artery disease.* J Am Coll Cardiol, 2005 **46**(9): p. 1643-8.
69. Henry, T.D., B.H. Annex, G.R. McKendall, et al., *The VIVA trial: Vascular endothelial growth factor in Ischemia for Vascular Angiogenesis.* Circulation, 2003. **107**(10): p. 1359-65.
70. Senti, S., M. Fleisch, M. Billinger, B. Meier, and C. Seiler, *Long-term physical exercise and quantitatively assessed human coronary collateral circulation.* J Am Coll Cardiol, 1998. **32**(1): p. 49-56.
71. Belardinelli, R., D. Georgiou, L. Ginzton, G. Cianci, and A. Purcaro, *Effects of moderate exercise training on thallium uptake and contractile response to low-dose dobutamine of dysfunctional myocardium in patients with ischemic cardiomyopathy.* Circulation, 1998. **97**(6): p. 553-61.
72. Niebauer, J., R. Hambrecht, C. Marburger, et al., *Impact of intensive physical exercise and low-fat diet on collateral vessel formation in stable angina pectoris and angiographically confirmed coronary artery disease.* Am J Cardiol, 1995. **76**(11): p. 771-5.
73. Zbinden, R., S. Zbinden, P. Meier, et al., *Coronary collateral flow in response to endurance exercise training.* Eur J Cardiovasc Prev Rehabil, 2007. **14**(2): p. 250-7.
74. Soroff, H.S., W.C. Birtwell, F. Giron, J.A. Collins, and R.A. Deterling, Jr., *Support of the systemic circulation and left ventricular assist by synchronous pulsation of extramural pressure.* Surg Forum, 1965. **16**: p. 148-50.
75. Giron, F., W.C. Birtwell, H.S. Soroff, et al., *Assisted circulation by synchronous pulsation of extramural pressure.* Surgery, 1966. **60**(4): p. 894-901.
76. Ruiz, U., H.S. Soroff, W.C. Birtwell, and R.A. Deterling, Jr., *External synchronous assisted circulation: experimental and clinical evaluation.* Surg Forum, 1968. **19**: p. 127-8.
77. Soroff, H.S., W.C. Birtwell, H.J. Levine, A.E. Bellas, and R.A. Deterling, Jr., *Effect of counterpulsation upon the myocardial oxygen consumption and heart work.* Surg Forum, 1962. **13**: p. 174-6.
78. Sachs, B.F., H.S. Soroff, W.C. Birtwell, H.J. Levine, and R.A. Deterling, Jr., *Hemodynamic effects of counterpulsation. Evaluation of proper and improper phasing on left ventricular oxygen consumption.* Tufts Folia Med, 1963. **9**: p. 17-22.
79. Birtwell, W.C., U. Ruiz, H.S. Soroff, D. DesMarais, and R.A. Deterling, Jr., *Technical considerations in the design of a clinical system for external left ventricular assist.* Trans Am Soc Artif Intern Organs, 1968. **14**: p. 304-10.
80. Mueller, H., *Are intra-aortic balloon pumping and external counterpulsation effective in the treatment of cardiogenic shock?* Cardiovasc Clin, 1977. **8**(1): p. 87-102.
81. Zheng, Z.S., T.M. Li, H. Kambic, et al., *Sequential external counterpulsation (SECP) in China.* Trans Am Soc Artif Intern Organs, 1983. **29**: p. 599-603.
82. FDA, U.S. *Products and Medical Procedures: Device Approvals and Clearences.* 2003 [cited 02.12.2009]; Available from: http://www.accessdata.fda.gov/cdrh_docs/pdf2/K023427.pdf.

83. Arora, R.R., T.M. Chou, D. Jain, et al., *The multicenter study of enhanced external counterpulsation (MUST-EECP): effect of EECP on exercise-induced myocardial ischemia and anginal episodes.* J Am Coll Cardiol, 1999. **33**(7): p. 1833-40.
84. Loh, P.H., J.G. Cleland, A.A. Louis, et al., *Enhanced External Counterpulsation in the Treatment of Chronic Refractory Angina: A Long-term Follow-up Outcome from the International Enhanced External Counterpulsation Patient Registry.* Clin Cardiol, 2008. **31**(4): p. 159-64.
85. Michaels, A.D., A. Raisinghani, O. Soran, et al., *The effects of enhanced external counterpulsation on myocardial perfusion in patients with stable angina: a multicenter radionuclide study.* Am Heart J, 2005. **150**(5): p. 1066-73.
86. Urano, H., H. Ikeda, T. Ueno, et al., *Enhanced external counterpulsation improves exercise tolerance, reduces exercise-induced myocardial ischemia and improves left ventricular diastolic filling in patients with coronary artery disease.* J Am Coll Cardiol, 2001. **37**(1): p. 93-9.
87. Tartaglia, J., J. Stenerson, Jr., R. Charney, et al., *Exercise capability and myocardial perfusion in chronic angina patients treated with enhanced external counterpulsation.* Clin Cardiol, 2003. **26**(6): p. 287-90.
88. Feldman, A.M., M.A. Silver, G.S. Francis, et al., *Enhanced external counterpulsation improves exercise tolerance in patients with chronic heart failure.* J Am Coll Cardiol, 2006. **48**(6): p. 1198-205.
89. Campbell, A.R., D. Satran, A.G. Zenovich, et al., *Enhanced external counterpulsation improves systolic blood pressure in patients with refractory angina.* Am Heart J, 2008. **156**(6): p. 1217-22.
90. Werner, D., P. Tragner, A. Wawer, et al., *Enhanced external counterpulsation: a new technique to augment renal function in liver cirrhosis.* Nephrol Dial Transplant, 2005. **20**(5): p. 920-6.
91. Rajaram, S.S., J. Shanahan, C. Ash, A.S. Walters, and G. Weisfogel, *Enhanced external counter pulsation (EECP) as a novel treatment for restless legs syndrome (RLS): a preliminary test of the vascular neurologic hypothesis for RLS.* Sleep Med, 2005. **6**(2): p. 101-6.
92. Froschermaier, S.E., D. Werner, S. Leike, et al., *Enhanced external counterpulsation as a new treatment modality for patients with erectile dysfunction.* Urol Int, 1998. **61**(3): p. 168-71.
93. Offergeld, C., D. Werner, M. Schneider, W.G. Daniel, and K.B. Huttenbrink, *[Pneumatic external counterpulsation (PECP): a new treatment option in therapy refractory inner ear disorders?].* Laryngorhinootologie, 2000. **79**(9): p. 503-9.
94. Han, J.H., T.W. Leung, W.W. Lam, et al., *Preliminary findings of external counterpulsation for ischemic stroke patient with large artery occlusive disease.* Stroke, 2008. **39**(4): p. 1340-3.
95. Michaels, A.D., E.D. Kennard, S.E. Kelsey, et al., *Does higher diastolic augmentation predict clinical benefit from enhanced external counterpulsation?: Data from the International EECP Patient Registry (IEPR).* Clin Cardiol, 2001. **24**(6): p. 453-8.
96. Lakshmi, M.V., E.D. Kennard, S.F. Kelsey, R. Holubkov, and A.D. Michaels, *Relation of the pattern of diastolic augmentation during a course of enhanced external counterpulsation (EECP) to clinical benefit (from the International EECP Patient Registry [IEPR]).* Am J Cardiol, 2002. **89**(11): p. 1303-5.

97. Stys, T., W.E. Lawson, J.C. Hui, et al., *Acute hemodynamic effects and angina improvement with enhanced external counterpulsation.* Angiology, 2001. **52**(10): p. 653-8.
98. Suresh, K., S. Simandl, W.E. Lawson, et al., *Maximizing the hemodynamic benefit of enhanced external counterpulsation.* Clin Cardiol, 1998. **21**(9): p. 649-53.
99. Michaels, A.D., P.A. McCullough, O.Z. Soran, et al., *Primer: practical approach to the selection of patients for and application of EECP.* Nat Clin Pract Cardiovasc Med, 2006. **3**(11): p. 623-32.
100. Bonetti, P.O., D.R. Holmes, Jr., A. Lerman, and G.W. Barsness, *Enhanced external counterpulsation for ischemic heart disease: what's behind the curtain?* J Am Coll Cardiol, 2003. **41**(11): p. 1918-25.
101. Michaels, A.D., M. Accad, T.A. Ports, and W. Grossman, *Left ventricular systolic unloading and augmentation of intracoronary pressure and Doppler flow during enhanced external counterpulsation.* Circulation, 2002. **106**(10): p. 1237-42.
102. Werner, D., F. Michalk, B. Hinz, et al., *Impact of enhanced external counterpulsation on peripheral circulation.* Angiology, 2007. **58**(2): p. 185-90.
103. Schaper, W. and D. Scholz, *Factors regulating arteriogenesis.* Arterioscler Thromb Vasc Biol, 2003. **23**(7): p. 1143-51.
104. Chatzizisis, Y.S., A.U. Coskun, M. Jonas, et al., *Role of endothelial shear stress in the natural history of coronary atherosclerosis and vascular remodeling: molecular, cellular, and vascular behavior.* J Am Coll Cardiol, 2007. **49**(25): p. 2379-93.
105. Mees, B., S. Wagner, E. Ninci, et al., *Endothelial nitric oxide synthase activity is essential for vasodilation during blood flow recovery but not for arteriogenesis.* Arterioscler Thromb Vasc Biol, 2007. **27**(9): p. 1926-33.
106. Jacobey, W.J.T., George T. Smith, Richard Gorlin, Dwight E. Harken, *A new therapeutic approach to acute coronary occlusion : II. Opening dormant coronary collateral channels by counterpulsation.* The American Journal of Cardiology, 1963. **11**(2): p. 218-227.
107. Rosensweig, J., C Borromeo, S. Chatterjee, N. Sheiner, and A. Mayman, *Treatment of coronary insufficiency by counterpulsation.* Ann Thorac Surg, 1966. **2**(5): p. 706-13.
108. Wu, G., Z. Du, C. Hu, et al., *Angiogenic effects of long-term enhanced external counterpulsation in a dog model of myocardial infarction.* Am J Physiol Heart Circ Physiol, 2006. **290**(1): p. H248-54.
109. Masuda, D., R. Nohara, T. Hirai, et al., *Enhanced external counterpulsation improved myocardial perfusion and coronary flow reserve in patients with chronic stable angina; evaluation by(13)N-ammonia positron emission tomography.* Eur Heart J, 2001. **22**(16): p. 1451-8.
110. Arora, R.R. and S. Bergmann, *Effects of enhanced external counterpulsation (EECP) on myocardial perfusion.* Am J Ther, 2007. **14**(6): p. 519-23.
111. Hutcheson, I.R. and T.M. Griffith, *Release of endothelium-derived relaxing factor is modulated both by frequency and amplitude of pulsatile flow.* Am J Physiol, 1991. **261**(1 Pt 2): p. H257-62.
112. Shechter, M., S. Matetzky, M.S. Feinberg, et al., *External counterpulsation therapy improves endothelial function in patients with refractory angina pectoris.* J Am Coll Cardiol, 2003. **42**(12): p. 2090-5.

113. Bonetti, P.O., G.W. Barsness, P.C. Keelan, et al., *Enhanced external counterpulsation improves endothelial function in patients with symptomatic coronary artery disease.* J Am Coll Cardiol, 2003. **41**(10): p. 1761-8.
114. Levenson, J., M.G. Pernollet, M.C. Iliou, M.A. Devynck, and A. Simon, *Cyclic GMP release by acute enhanced external counterpulsation.* Am J Hypertens, 2006. **19**(8): p. 867-72.
115. Akhtar, M., G.F. Wu, Z.M. Du, Z.S. Zheng, and A.D. Michaels, *Effect of external counterpulsation on plasma nitric oxide and endothelin-1 levels.* Am J Cardiol, 2006. **98**(1): p. 28-30.
116. Tao, J., C. Tu, Z. Yang, et al., *Enhanced external counterpulsation improves endothelium-dependent vasorelaxation in the carotid arteries of hypercholesterolemic pigs.* Int J Cardiol, 2006. **112**(3): p. 269-74.
117. Nichols, W.W., J.C. Estrada, R.W. Braith, K. Owens, and C.R. Conti, *Enhanced external counterpulsation treatment improves arterial wall properties and wave reflection characteristics in patients with refractory angina.* J Am Coll Cardiol, 2006. **48**(6): p. 1208-14.
118. Saito, M., H. Okayama, K. Nishimura, et al., *Possible link between large artery stiffness and coronary flow velocity reserve.* Heart, 2008. **94**(6): p. e20.
119. Lawson, W.E., J.C. Hui, H.S. Soroff, et al., *Efficacy of enhanced external counterpulsation in the treatment of angina pectoris.* Am J Cardiol, 1992. **70**(9): p. 859-62.
120. Lawson, W.E., J.C. Hui, Z.S. Zheng, et al., *Can angiographic findings predict which coronary patients will benefit from enhanced external counterpulsation?* Am J Cardiol, 1996. **77**(12): p. 1107-9.
121. Lawson, W.E., J.C. Hui, T. Guo, L. Burger, and P.F. Cohn, *Prior revascularization increases the effectiveness of enhanced external counterpulsation.* Clin Cardiol, 1998. **21**(11): p. 841-4.
122. Stys, T.P., W.E. Lawson, J.C. Hui, et al., *Effects of enhanced external counterpulsation on stress radionuclide coronary perfusion and exercise capacity in chronic stable angina pectoris.* Am J Cardiol, 2002. **89**(7): p. 822-4.
123. Bagger, J.P., R.J. Hall, G. Koutroulis, and P. Nihoyannopoulos, *Effect of enhanced external counterpulsation on dobutamine-induced left ventricular wall motion abnormalities in severe chronic angina pectoris.* Am J Cardiol, 2004. **93**(4): p. 465-7.
124. Novo, G., J.P. Bagger, R. Carta, et al., *Enhanced external counterpulsation for treatment of refractory angina pectoris.* J Cardiovasc Med (Hagerstown), 2006. **7**(5): p. 335-9.
125. Dockery, F., C. Rajkumar, C.J. Bulpitt, R.J. Hall, and J.P. Bagger, *Enhanced external counterpulsation does not alter arterial stiffness in patients with angina.* Clin Cardiol, 2004. **27**(12): p. 689-92.
126. Hasdai, D., R.J. Gibbons, D.R. Holmes, Jr., S.T. Higano, and A. Lerman, *Coronary endothelial dysfunction in humans is associated with myocardial perfusion defects.* Circulation, 1997. **96**(10): p. 3390-5.
127. Kronhaus, K.D. and W.E. Lawson, *Enhanced external counterpulsation is an effective treatment for Syndrome X.* Int J Cardiol, 2008.
128. Bonetti, P.O., S.N. Gadasalli, A. Lerman, and G.W. Barsness, *Successful treatment of symptomatic coronary endothelial dysfunction with enhanced external counterpulsation.* Mayo Clin Proc, 2004. **79**(5): p. 690-2.

129. Lee, C.M., Y.W. Wu, H.Y. Jui, et al., *Enhanced external counterpulsation reduces lung/heart ratio at stress in patients with coronary artery disease.* Cardiology, 2006. **106**(4): p. 237-40.
130. Kurata, C., K. Tawarahara, T. Taguchi, et al., *Lung thallium-201 uptake during exercise emission computed tomography.* J Nucl Med, 1991. **32**(3): p. 417-23.
131. Estahbanaty, G., N. Samiei, M. Maleki, et al., *Echocardiographic characteristics including tissue Doppler imaging after enhanced external counterpulsation therapy.* Am Heart Hosp J, 2007. **5**(4): p. 241-6.
132. Kumar, A., W.S. Aronow, A. Vadnerkar, et al., *Effect of enhanced external counterpulsation on clinical symptoms, quality of life, 6-minute walking distance, and echocardiographic measurements of left ventricular systolic and diastolic function after 35 days of treatment and at 1-year follow up in 47 patients with chronic refractory angina pectoris.* Am J Ther, 2009. **16**(2): p. 116-8.
133. Michaels, A.D., B.A. Bart, T. Pinto, et al., *The effects of enhanced external counterpulsation on time- and frequency-domain measures of heart rate variability.* J Electrocardiol, 2007.
134. Tsuji, H., F.J. Venditti, Jr., E.S. Manders, et al., *Determinants of heart rate variability.* J Am Coll Cardiol, 1996. **28**(6): p. 1539-46.
135. Ryan, T.J., W.B. Bauman, J.W. Kennedy, et al., *Guidelines for percutaneous transluminal coronary angioplasty. A report of the American Heart Association/American College of Cardiology Task Force on Assessment of Diagnostic and Therapeutic Cardiovascular Procedures (Committee on Percutaneous Transluminal Coronary Angioplasty).* Circulation, 1993. **88**(6): p. 2987-3007.
136. Ryan, T.J., F.J. Klocke, and W.A. Reynolds, *Clinical competence in percutaneous transluminal coronary angioplasty. A statement for physicians from the ACP/ACC/AHA Task Force on Clinical Privileges in Cardiology.* J Am Coll Cardiol, 1990. **15**(7): p. 1469-74.
137. Gibbons, R.J., J. Abrams, K. Chatterjee, et al., *ACC/AHA 2002 guideline update for the management of patients with chronic stable angina--summary article: a report of the American College of Cardiology/American Heart Association Task Force on practice guidelines (Committee on the Management of Patients With Chronic Stable Angina).* J Am Coll Cardiol, 2003. **41**(1): p. 159-68.
138. Pijls, N.H., B. De Bruyne, K. Peels, et al., *Measurement of fractional flow reserve to assess the functional severity of coronary-artery stenoses.* N Engl J Med, 1996. **334**(26): p. 1703-8.
139. Billinger, M., L. Raeber, C. Seiler, et al., *Coronary collateral perfusion in patients with coronary artery disease: effect of metoprolol.* Eur Heart J, 2004. **25**(7): p. 565-70.
140. Egstrup, K. and P.E. Andersen, Jr., *Transient myocardial ischemia during nifedipine therapy in stable angina pectoris, and its relation to coronary collateral flow and comparison with metoprolol.* Am J Cardiol, 1993. **71**(2): p. 177-83.
141. Cohn, P.F., *Effects of calcium channel blockers on the coronary circulation.* Am J Hypertens, 1990. **3**(12 Pt 2): p. 299S-304S.
142. Magrini, F., M. Shimizu, N. Roberts, et al., *Converting-enzyme inhibition and coronary blood flow.* Circulation, 1987. **75**(1 Pt 2): p. I168-74.

143. Joffe, H.V., R.Y. Kwong, M.D. Gerhard-Herman, et al., *Beneficial effects of eplerenone versus hydrochlorothiazide on coronary circulatory function in patients with diabetes mellitus.* J Clin Endocrinol Metab, 2007. **92**(7): p. 2552-8.

144. Dincer, I., A. Ongun, S. Turhan, et al., *Association between the dosage and duration of statin treatment with coronary collateral development.* Coron Artery Dis, 2006. **17**(6): p. 561-5.

145. Pourati, I., C. Kimmelstiel, W. Rand, and R.H. Karas, *Statin use is associated with enhanced collateralization of severely diseased coronary arteries.* Am Heart J, 2003. **146**(5): p. 876-81.

146. Bech, G.J., B. De Bruyne, N.H. Pijls, et al., *Fractional flow reserve to determine the appropriateness of angioplasty in moderate coronary stenosis: a randomized trial.* Circulation, 2001. **103**(24): p. 2928-34.

147. Trappe, H.J. and H. Lollgen, *[Guidelines for ergometry. German Society of Cardiology--Heart and Cardiovascular Research].* Z Kardiol, 2000. **89**(9): p. 821-31.

148. Pijls, N.H., J.A. van Son, R.L. Kirkeeide, B. De Bruyne, and K.L. Gould, *Experimental basis of determining maximum coronary, myocardial, and collateral blood flow by pressure measurements for assessing functional stenosis severity before and after percutaneous transluminal coronary angioplasty.* Circulation, 1993. **87**(4): p. 1354-67.

149. Pijls, N.H., B. Van Gelder, P. Van der Voort, et al., *Fractional flow reserve. A useful index to evaluate the influence of an epicardial coronary stenosis on myocardial blood flow.* Circulation, 1995. **92**(11): p. 3183-93.

150. Nico H. J. Pijls, B.d.B., *Coronary pressure, Chapter 12.5.2-12.5.5, page 251,.* 2000: Kluwer Academic Publishers.

151. De Bruyne, B. and J. Sarma, *Fractional flow reserve: a review: invasive imaging.* Heart, 2008. **94**(7): p. 949-59.

152. Bartunek, J., T.H. Marwick, A.C. Rodrigues, et al., *Dobutamine-induced wall motion abnormalities: correlations with myocardial fractional flow reserve and quantitative coronary angiography.* J Am Coll Cardiol, 1996. **27**(6): p. 1429-36.

153. Kern, M.J., A. Lerman, J.W. Bech, et al., *Physiological assessment of coronary artery disease in the cardiac catheterization laboratory: a scientific statement from the American Heart Association Committee on Diagnostic and Interventional Cardiac Catheterization, Council on Clinical Cardiology.* Circulation, 2006. **114**(12): p. 1321-41.

154. Pijls, N.H., *Is it time to measure fractional flow reserve in all patients?* J Am Coll Cardiol, 2003. **41**(7): p. 1122-4.

155. Pijls, N.H., P. van Schaardenburgh, G. Manoharan, et al., *Percutaneous coronary intervention of functionally nonsignificant stenosis: 5-year follow-up of the DEFER Study.* J Am Coll Cardiol, 2007. **49**(21): p. 2105-11.

156. Jones, C.J., L. Kuo, M.J. Davis, and W.M. Chilian, *Distribution and control of coronary microvascular resistance.* Adv Exp Med Biol, 1993. **346**: p. 181-8.

157. Camici, P.G. and F. Crea, *Coronary microvascular dysfunction.* N Engl J Med, 2007. **356**(8): p. 830-40.

158. De Bruyne, B., N.H. Pijls, L. Smith, M. Wievegg, and G.R. Heyndrickx, *Coronary thermodilution to assess flow reserve: experimental validation.* Circulation, 2001. **104**(17): p. 2003-6.

159. Pijls, N.H., B. De Bruyne, L. Smith, et al., *Coronary thermodilution to assess flow reserve: validation in humans.* Circulation, 2002. **105**(21): p. 2482-6.
160. McGinn, A.L., C.W. White, and R.F. Wilson, *Interstudy variability of coronary flow reserve. Influence of heart rate, arterial pressure, and ventricular preload* Circulation, 1990. **81**(4): p. 1319-30.
161. Kern, M.J., *Coronary physiology revisited : practical insights from the cardiac catheterization laboratory.* Circulation, 2000. **101**(11): p. 1344-51.
162. Aarnoudse, W., W.F. Fearon, G. Manoharan, et al., *Epicardial Stenosis Severity Does Not Affect Minimal Microcirculatory Resistance.* Circulation, 2004. **110**(15): p. 2137-2142.
163. Fearon, W.F., L.B. Balsam, H.M. Farouque, et al., *Novel index for invasively assessing the coronary microcirculation.* Circulation, 2003. **107**(25): p. 3129-32.
164. Aarnoudse, W., P. van den Berg, F. van de Vosse, et al., *Myocardial resistance assessed by guidewire-based pressure-temperature measurement: in vitro validation.* Catheter Cardiovasc Interv, 2004. **62**(1): p. 56-63.
165. Pijls, N.H., G.J. Uijen, A. Hoevelaken, et al., *Mean transit time for the assessment of myocardial perfusion by videodensitometry.* Circulation, 1990. **81**(4): p. 1331-40.
166. De Bruyne, B., N.H. Pijls, E. Barbato, et al., *Intracoronary and intravenous adenosine 5'-triphosphate, adenosine, papaverine, and contrast medium to assess fractional flow reserve in humans.* Circulation, 2003. **107**(14): p. 1877-83.
167. Masuda, D., M. Fujita, R. Nohara, A. Matsumori, and S. Sasayama, *Improvement of oxygen metabolism in ischemic myocardium as a result of enhanced external counterpulsation with heparin pretreatment for patients with stable angina.* Heart Vessels, 2004. **19**(2): p. 59-62.
168. Dahl, J.v., *Assessment of myocardial perfusion using cardiac positron emission tomography.* Z Kardiol, 2001. **90**(11): p. 835-847.
169. Garza, D., A.V. Tosh, R. Roberti, et al., *Detection of coronary collaterals using dipyridamole PET myocardial perfusion imaging with rubidium-82.* J Nucl Med, 1997. **38**(1): p. 39-43.
170. Sipahi, I., E.M. Tuzcu, P. Schoenhagen, et al., *Effects of normal, pre-hypertensive, and hypertensive blood pressure levels on progression of coronary atherosclerosis.* J Am Coll Cardiol, 2006. **48**(4): p. 833-8.
171. Burch, G.E., *Digital Plethysmography.* 1954, New York: Grune & Stratton Inc.
172. Zhang, Y., X. He, X. Chen, et al., *Enhanced external counterpulsation inhibits intimal hyperplasia by modifying shear stress responsive gene expression in hypercholesterolemic pigs.* Circulation, 2007. **116**(5): p. 526-34.
173. Vita, J.A. and G.F. Mitchell, *Effects of shear stress and flow pulsatility on endothelial function: insights gleaned from external counterpulsation therapy.* J Am Coll Cardiol, 2003. **42**(12): p. 2096-8.
174. Lawson, W.E., J.C. Hui, E.D. Kennard, G. Barsness, and S.F. Kelsey, *Predictors of benefit in angina patients one year after completing enhanced external counterpulsation: initial responders to treatment versus nonresponders.* Cardiology, 2005. **103**(4): p. 201-6.
175. Hemingway, H., C. Langenberg, J. Damant, et al., *Prevalence of angina in women versus men: a systematic review and meta-analysis of international variations across 31 countries.* Circulation, 2008. **117**(12): p. 1526-36.

176. Pepine, C.J., R.A. Kerensky, C.R. Lambert, et al., *Some thoughts on the vasculopathy of women with ischemic heart disease.* J Am Coll Cardiol, 2006. **47**(3 Suppl): p. S30-5.
177. Bittner, V., *Angina pectoris: reversal of the gender gap.* Circulation, 2008. **117**(12): p. 1505-7.
178. Cohn, P.F., *Enhanced external counterpulsation for the treatment of angina pectoris.* Prog Cardiovasc Dis, 2006. **49**(2): p. 88-97.
179. Crisafulli, A., F. Melis, F. Tocco, et al., *Exercise-induced and nitroglycerin-induced myocardial preconditioning improves hemodynamics in patients with angina.* Am J Physiol Heart Circ Physiol, 2004. **287**(1): p. H235-42.
180. Jneid, H., M. Chandra, M. Alshaher, et al., *Delayed preconditioning-mimetic actions of nitroglycerin in patients undergoing exercise tolerance tests.* Circulation, 2005. **111**(20): p. 2565-71.
181. Schaper, W., *The Collateral Circulation of the Heart.* 1971, New York: American Elsevier Publishing Company.
182. Pagonas, N., W. Utz, J. Schulz-Menger, et al., *Assessment of the effect of external counterpulsation on myocardial adaptive arteriogenesis by invasive functional measurements - design of the arteriogenesis network trial 2.* Int J Cardiol, 2009.
183. Buschmann, E.E., W. Utz, N. Pagonas, et al., *Improvement of fractional flow reserve and collateral flow by treatment with external counterpulsation (Art.Net.-2 Trial).* Eur J Clin Invest, 2009.
184. Gloekler, S., P. Meier, S.F. de Marchi, et al., *Coronary Collateral Growth by External Counterpulsation: A Randomized Controlled Trial.* Heart, 2009.
185. Carrao, A.C., W.M. Chilian, J. Yun, et al., *Stimulation of coronary collateral growth by granulocyte stimulating factor: role of reactive oxygen species.* Arterioscler Thromb Vasc Biol, 2009. **29**(11): p. 1817-22.
186. Buschmann, I.R., I.E. Hoefer, N. van Royen, et al., *GM-CSF: a strong arteriogenic factor acting by amplification of monocyte function.* Atherosclerosis, 2001. **159**(2): p. 343-56.
187. Bonetti, P.O., G.M. Pumper, S.T. Higano, et al., *Noninvasive identification of patients with early coronary atherosclerosis by assessment of digital reactive hyperemia.* J Am Coll Cardiol, 2004. **44**(11): p. 2137-41.
188. Hambrecht, R., A. Wolf, S. Gielen, et al., *Effect of exercise on coronary endothelial function in patients with coronary artery disease.* N Engl J Med, 2000. **342**(7): p. 454-60.
189. Wilkinson, I.B., A. Qasem, C.M. McEniery, et al., *Nitric Oxide Regulates Local Arterial Distensibility In Vivo.* Circulation, 2002. **105**(2): p. 213-217.
190. Pupita, G., A. Maseri, J.C. Kaski, et al., *Myocardial ischemia caused by distal coronary-artery constriction in stable angina pectoris.* N Engl J Med, 1990. **323**(8): p. 514-20.
191. Prati, F., T. Pawlowski, R. Gil, et al., *Stenting of culprit lesions in unstable angina leads to a marked reduction in plaque burden: a major role of plaque embolization? A serial intravascular ultrasound study.* Circulation, 2003. **107**(18): p. 2320-5.
192. Uren, N.G., T. Crake, D.C. Lefroy, et al., *Delayed recovery of coronary resistive vessel function after coronary angioplasty.* J Am Coll Cardiol, 1993. **21**(3): p. 612-21.
193. Ng, M.K.C., A.C. Yeung, and W.F. Fearon, *Invasive Assessment of the Coronary Microcirculation: Superior Reproducibility and Less Hemodynamic Dependence of*

Index of Microcirculatory Resistance Compared With Coronary Flow Reserve. Circulation, 2006. **113**(17): p. 2054-2061.
194. Karamitsos, T.D., J.M. Francis, S. Myerson, J.B. Selvanayagam, and S. Neubauer, *The role of cardiovascular magnetic resonance imaging in heart failure.* J Am Coll Cardiol, 2009. **54**(15): p. 1407-24.
195. Bellenger, N.G., F. Grothues, G.C. Smith, and D.J. Pennell, *Quantification of right and left ventricular function by cardiovascular magnetic resonance.* Herz, 2000. **25**(4): p. 392-9.
196. Esmaeilzadeh, M., A. Khaledifar, M. Maleki, et al., *Evaluation of left ventricular systolic and diastolic regional function after enhanced external counter pulsation therapy using strain rate imaging.* Eur J Echocardiogr, 2009. **10**(1): p. 120-6.
197. Levenson, J., A. Simon, J.L. Megnien, et al., *Effects of Enhanced External Counterpulsation on Carotid Circulation in Patients with Coronary Artery Disease.* Cardiology, 2006 **108**(2): p. 104-110.
198. Kaptchuk, T.J., P. Goldman, D.A. Stone, and W.B. Stason, *Do medical devices have enhanced placebo effects?* J Clin Epidemiol, 2000. **53**(8): p. 786-92.

7 Appendix

7.1 List of abbreviations

ACE	angiotensin converting enzyme
AHA	American Heart Association
BMI	body mass index
bpm	beats per minute
CABG	coronary artery bypass graft
CAD	coronary artery disease
CCS	Canadian Cardiovascular Society
CFIp	pressure-derived collateral flow index
CFIv	velocity-derived collateral flow index
CMR	cardiac magnetic resonance
D/S ratio	diastolic to systolic augmentation ratio
ECG	electrocardiography
ECP	external counterpulsation
EECP	enhanced external counterpulsation
FFR	fractional flow reserve
GM-CSF	granulocyte-macrophage colony-stimulating factor
HDL	high density lipoprotein
IEPR	international enhanced external counterpulsation patient registry
IHD	ischemic heart disease
IMR	index of microcirculatory resistance
IMRcor	IMR corrected for the coronary occlusion pressure

IMRcvp	IMR corrected for the central venous pressure
LDL	low density lipoprotein
LV	left ventricle
LVEF	left ventricular ejection fraction
LVEDP	left ventricular end diastolic pressure
MI	myocardial infarction
NSTE-ACS	Non ST-segment elevation acute coronary syndrome
NYHA	New York Heart Association
Pa	mean aortic pressure
PCI	percutaneous coronary intervention
Pd	mean distal coronary pressure
PET	positron emission tomography
PTCA	percutaneous transluminal coronary angioplasty
Pv	mean central venous pressure
Pw	mean distal coronary pressure during balloon occlusion (coronary wedge pressure)
Rcoll	collateral resistance index
SD	standard deviation
SE	standard error
SPECT	Single Photon Emission Computed Tomography
STE-ACS	ST-segment elevation acute coronary syndrome
STEMI	ST-segment elevation myocardial infarction
Voccl	flow velocity during vessel occlusion
Vpat	flow velocity during vessel patency

7.2 Acknnowledgments

I would like to thank PD Dr. Ivo Buschmann for kindly providing the interesting theme, and the always reliable supervision. My very special thanks to Dr. Eva Buschman for our excellent cooperation in all phases of the study and for her constructive advice in handling this theme.

I also thank Prof. L. Thierfelder for the co-supervision of PhD and for the realization of the study at the Franz Volhard Clinic. I am grateful to PD Dr. M. Gross and the staff of the cardiac catheterization laboratories for performing the invasive measurements. I would like also to thank the working group for cardiovascular MRI at the Franz Volhard Clinic for the introduction into cardiac MRI, and for helping in evaluating the images.

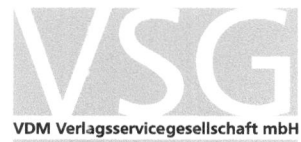

Die VDM Verlagsservicegesellschaft sucht für wissenschaftliche Verlage abgeschlossene und herausragende

Dissertationen, Habilitationen, Diplomarbeiten, Master Theses, Magisterarbeiten usw.

für die kostenlose Publikation als Fachbuch.

Sie verfügen über eine Arbeit, die hohen inhaltlichen und formalen Ansprüchen genügt, und haben Interesse an einer honorarvergüteten Publikation?

Dann senden Sie bitte erste Informationen über sich und Ihre Arbeit per Email an *info@vdm-vsg.de*.

Sie erhalten kurzfristig unser Feedback!

VDM Verlagsservicegesellschaft mbH
Dudweiler Landstr. 99　　　　　　　Telefon +49 681 3720 174
D - 66123 Saarbrücken　　　　　　　Fax　　　+49 681 3720 1749
www.vdm-vsg.de

Die VDM Verlagsservicegesellschaft mbH vertritt

 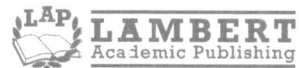 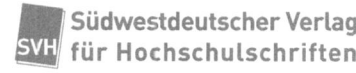

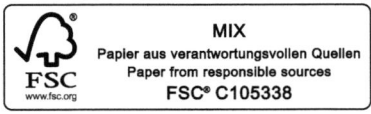

Printed by Books on Demand GmbH, Norderstedt / Germany